Art & Makeup

Author's dedication:
To Brendan and Eva Marie Grealis

Published in 2015
by Laurence King Publishing Ltd
361–373 City Road
London EC1V 1LR
Tel +44 20 7841 6900
Fax +44 20 7841 6910
E enquiries@laurenceking.com
www.laurenceking.com

www.lan-makeup.com

Co-written and edited by Hannah Kane
Creative Direction & Makeup: Lan Nguyen-Grealis
Fashion Director: Karl Willett
Cover image: Leila wearing Justin Smith Esquire;
photograph Camille Sanson
Special thanks to Kryolan for their support and to
Disciple Productions
www.disciple-productions.com

A catalogue record for this book is available from
the British Library

ISBN 978 178067 485 8
Designed by Charlotte Klingholz
Project Editor: Gaynor Sermon
Printed in China

Art & Makeup

Lan Nguyen-Grealis

Laurence King Publishing

Contents

Foreword

by Rankin

The relationship between a photographer and makeup artist is one of the most important aspects of any fashion or beauty shoot. For me, I'm looking for artists who give me creative traction, people I can bounce ideas off and who inspire me to push my photography as much as I give them the space to push their own work. It isn't simply about craft but imagination, concepts and creative ambitions that take you beyond, into an artistry that is unlike any other discipline.

I'm fortunate enough to have worked with Lan and seen the excellence of her work. What I love about this book is that it offers a unique insight into her inspiration and in turn her process. It reminds us that our understanding of techniques begins with history, art, culture, and all the wider things that inspire us, but can get forgotten along the way. It is these broader strokes that will empower you to take the finer ones.

Art

Mak

& *ceup*

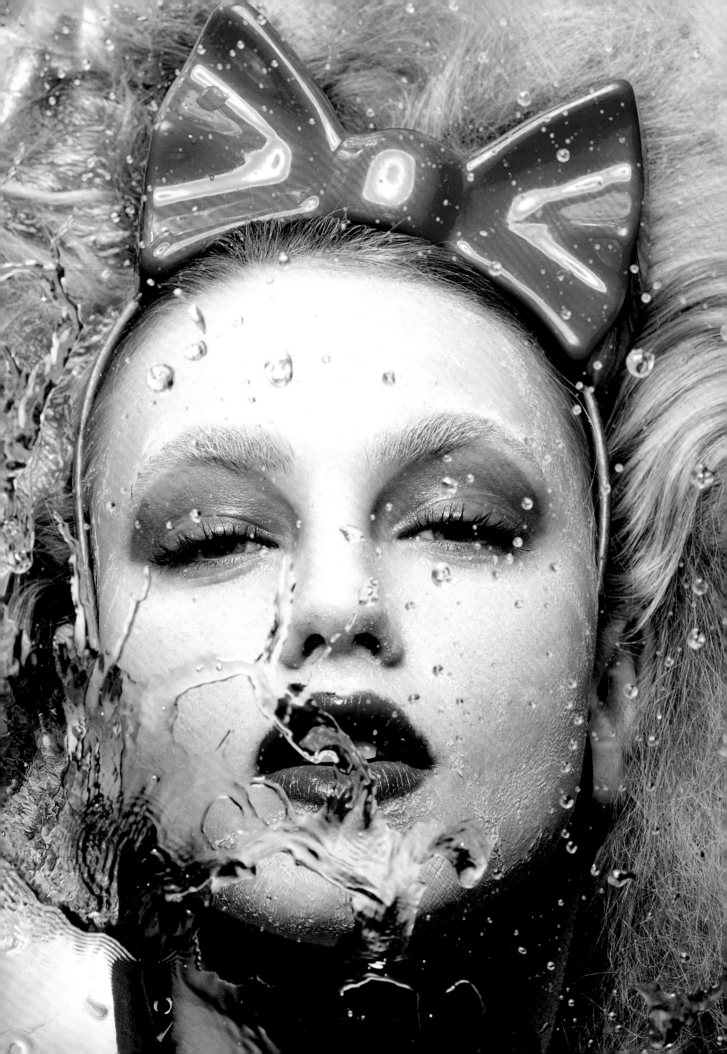

Prologue

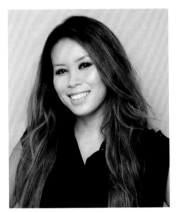

Lan Nguyen-Grealis is the youngest Golden Mask award winner (2013) for Makeup Art, and National Professional UK Makeup Awards Winner (2011) for Best Studio Makeup, and Overall Winner.

Originally self-taught, Lan brings to the world of makeup her unique flair and knowledge of art techniques, creating avant-garde looks and stunning beauty editorials for fashion, music and film. Now, with more than a decade of experience, Lan continues to enjoy a rewarding career designing iconic looks for leading fashion show designers.

Lan is the magic ingredient in many a celebrity's styling team, and shares her knowledge through teaching students across the globe.

Makeup Kryolan Supracolor 079, Icicle Gel,
Thickening Agent; MAC Lipstick (Lady
Danger) **Photography** Camille Sanson
Headpiece Justin Smith **Hair** Jose Quijano
using Catwalk by TIGI **Model** Karina White
Makeup Assistant Alexa Taylor
Photography Assistant Indigo Rohrer

Below and middle This is the mechanical heart that I designed for an Alexandra Palace fireworks night special. Our art class was commissioned by the local council to design something for their lighthouse sculpture, which was over 3 m tall. **Bottom** June 1998. This is my A-level presentation of artwork, for which I received the highest grade. It was based on Renoir, Cézanne and some famous architects.

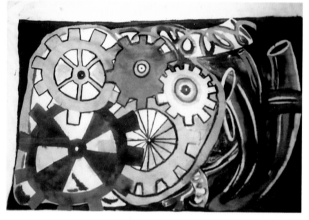

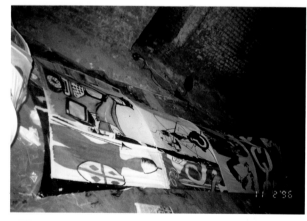

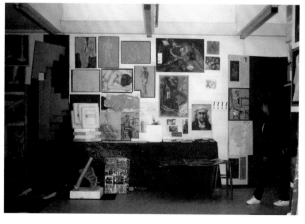

The early years

Born on 4 March 1980 in Dublin, Ireland, I was one of the first Irish-born children of the Vietnamese boat people who were helped by Irish missionaries in 1979. My parents were only in their late teens when they decided to settle with the help of the Irish government. Named 'Ailan' after the country and town I was born in, I grew up travelling on the road until we settled in a town called Waterford – famous for its crystal. My parents worked at the factory etching mirrors and cutting crystal, and watching them work inspired my creativity at a young age.

I displayed an aptitude for drawing as a child, and winning a drawing competition at school fuelled my dreams of becoming an artist. I would often be told that I should get a real job as a doctor, lawyer, teacher or even a musician – anything but an artist! Or marry a rich man ... in keeping with tradition in the Vietnamese culture at this time. This was probably the catalyst that drove me to succeed.

Luckily for me, my friends, teachers, and people around me understood my need to be creative and would offer positive feedback and encouragement. I would escape my five other siblings, cycle to the beaches and lay under big skies, dreaming of one day making it big and proving everyone wrong.

I attended Presentation Convent, an all-girls primary school. I learnt about Mother Teresa, whom I admired for making such a big difference in the world – she inspired me to think big. I also wanted to be an artist like my heroes Picasso and Rembrandt. I loved dressing up every day for school and it was a ritual to prepare my hair the night before each school day. Curling, cutting or just setting it in rags for the next day, I would spend hours playing with ideas. I also loved watching my cousins getting ready each day with their perfect '80s quiffs and the ever-present smell of Elnett hairspray. Although no makeup was

'I would often be told that I should get a real job as a doctor, lawyer, teacher or even a musician – anything but an artist! Or marry a rich man ... in keeping with tradition in the Vietnamese culture at this time. This was probably the catalyst that drove me to succeed.'

'At every opportunity my mother would apply mascara and lipstick on me – which at the time I hated with a passion.'

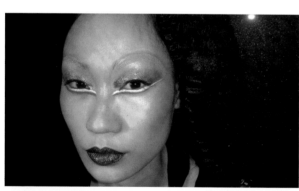

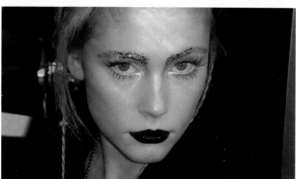

allowed at school, at every opportunity my mother would apply mascara and lipstick on me – which at the time I hated with a passion!

The big city
Moving to London in 1992 was a huge culture shock – everything was so big – but it was also a great opportunity for adventure. Art was my comfort zone and I stayed after school hours on many occasions and did extra classes in life drawing. I also enjoyed teaching the younger students the importance of art. While others left school to do 'real' work, I stayed on to study art, still unsure of what my future would be. At Middlesex University I did a foundation course in Art and Design, experiencing the different aspects of photography, design, sculpture, fine art, and textiles. I discovered I had a love for textiles, which led me to Central Saint Martins, one of the most prestigious fashion colleges in the world, to study Fashion Design with Marketing. I loved the idea of fashion, but all of a sudden it became a chore and not a hobby. The mechanics of design and pattern cutting made me very impatient, as I loved the idea

Opposite, top My first 'off-schedule' London Fashion Week show for designer Bernard Chandran, where I was key makeup artist.
Bottom One of my favourite avant-garde designers, Inbar Spector, was a dream to work with, and always pushed boundaries with her work.

This page, below left and right This was our small syndication team, working in Paris for German *Cosmopolitan.* Included is photographer Steve Wood.

Bottom Watching a Valentino couture show in Paris; this picture was taken with my disposable camera.

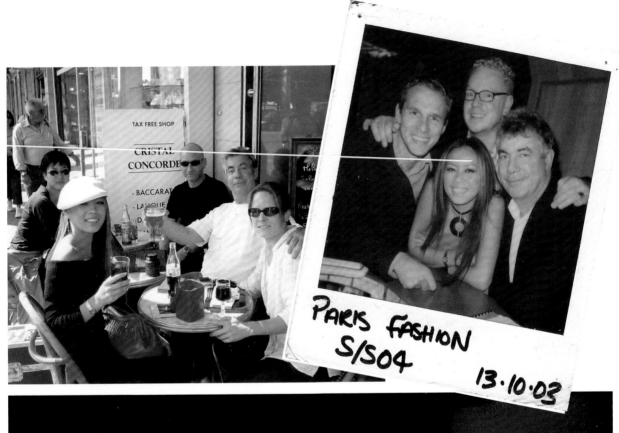

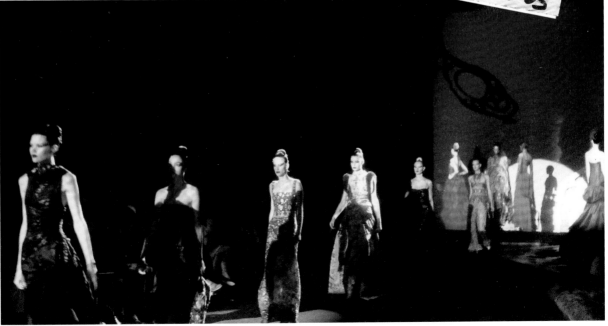

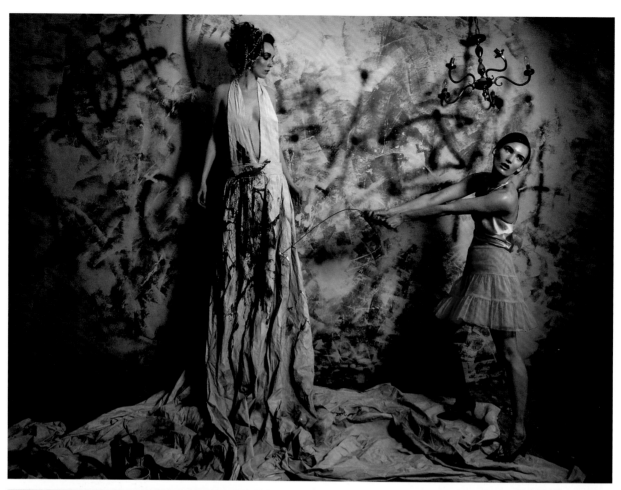

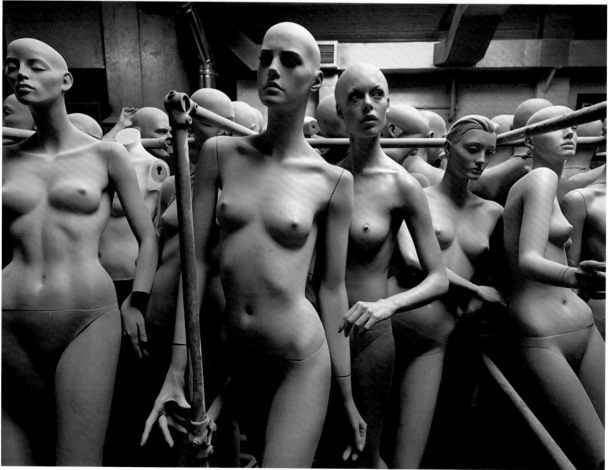

Opposite, top This was my first collaboration with photographer Camille Sanson, using MAC cosmetics. I was very proud of it.

Opposite, bottom A photoshoot for Rootstein mannequins, which was my first time using special effects products, by Kryolan. **Photography** Roger Mavity.

Below This collection of mannequins was for fashion designer Sorapol's S/S14 collection launch at the Serpentine Gallery, London.

'I'm fascinated by how hard it becomes to distinguish, in modern life, between truth and falsehood, spin and substance. Mannequins seem to me to be the perfect metaphor for this confusion - they are in the same moment so lifelike and yet so lifeless.'

– Roger Mavity, photographer

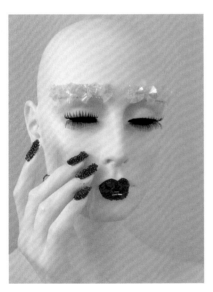
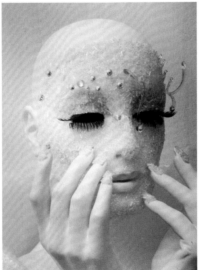
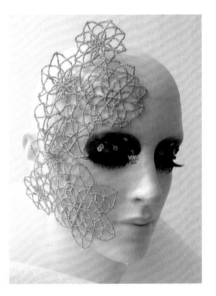

of making rather than working out design patterns that involved a lot of maths. Still not knowing where it would take me, I carried on for three years.

Luck of the Irish
During my final year of study in the summer of 2002 something that I couldn't have predicted happened. I had been working on my final project continuously for days when I left the room for a break – I heard a loud bang and ran to see what had happened. No words can describe how unfortunate and unlucky I felt when I saw that the whole ceiling had collapsed and destroyed everything I had been working on. It was all lost in the rubble forever.

Making it up as I went along
I had been working in PR at the time to pay for my fees, and stumbled upon an opportunity to work at a photographic studio right in the heart of London, where I became a coffee girl and was introduced to the world of makeup art. This is where it all began. One day they were short-staffed, so they asked me to fill in. I was given a set of brushes and sent on my way to do makeup for their customers. I was so worried that I wouldn't get it right but threw myself into it anyway and, putting their needs first, I completed the day without any hiccups. For three years I never stopped …

Show time
… until a chance meeting with a photographer called Steve Wood, who invited me to do a shoot with him and one of his important clients. I did so well that he offered me a job assisting him during London Fashion Week and I jumped at the chance. This was where my eyes were opened to the real world of fashion and

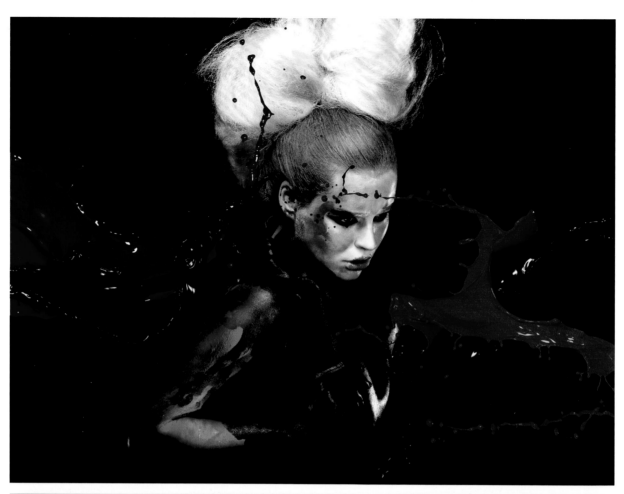

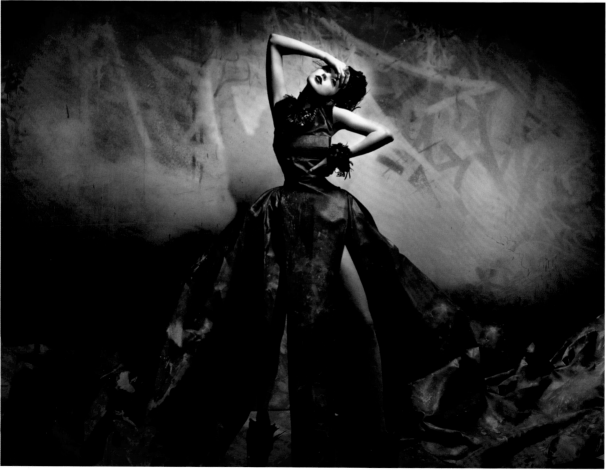

Opposite, top One of my first experimental photoshoots using paints and greasepaint from Kryolan. **Photography** Camille Sanson.

Opposite, bottom I was approached to collaborate with the graffiti artist known as Edge to develop an image that represented fashion. The dress was a collaboration with fashion stylist Shyla Hassan and photographer Camille Sanson. Once made, Edge spray-painted and worked on his graffiti design. Edge also designed the colours and backdrop, and I developed the concept of the doll-like model in 1920s' couture.

'I worked with all kinds of clientele, no job was too small for me, and I often did unpaid work, believing it was a learning tool.'

I saw how the whole industry took shape. During Paris Couture Fashion Week 2003 I met the legendary makeup artist Pat McGrath doing makeup backstage at Dior. It was a turning point to see how she demonstrated her flawless techniques on Alek Wek with her signature ruby crystal lips.

There are moments backstage that should not be spoken about, and I quickly learnt the etiquette – be discreet. There is an unspoken respect for the designer and team involved in order for a show to run smoothly. I knew that I had found a place for myself backstage – for the first time in my life I knew this was a place I could call home. I spent three years travelling to New York, Milan, Paris and London Fashion Weeks, season after season, working hard with Steve Wood as his photography assistant and runner. My job included interviewing all the next top models and dealing with press enquiries, editing images for the magazines and fighting to get a good position in the photographers' pit.

In the course of my travels I met fashion icons such as the late Alexander McQueen, Dennis Hopper and Tom Ford, to name but a few. Suddenly, there I was, holding a camera for Mario Testino, having a conversation with Shaggy or Paris Hilton or André Leon Talley, working for *Vogue* at the time. I wish I could go back to that period with what I know now and utilize my time properly, but I was young and naïve. I was probably most star-struck meeting Oprah and the First Lady. The stories will live with me forever as my secret, but for now I am so thankful to have had that opportunity.

Going solo
Deciding to go freelance was a tough decision because I had no assisting experience and no mentor to guide me, not to mention no job security or guarantee of money. Countless knocking on agency doors led to false promises that one day I may get a call. It was a very disheartening time, and I thought to myself that 'maybe it wasn't meant to be', but something inside me wanted to carry on. What I did have were a few trusted friends who were makeup artists and they encouraged me to keep going. I applied for any job where I could get makeup experience and, from there, word of mouth spread. I tested with many new

Working with movement and loose powders by
Kryolan. I used pink powder pigment and built
up the colour to fall from the model's hands,
creating graduated colour on the dress and on
her body. **Photography** Camille Sanson.

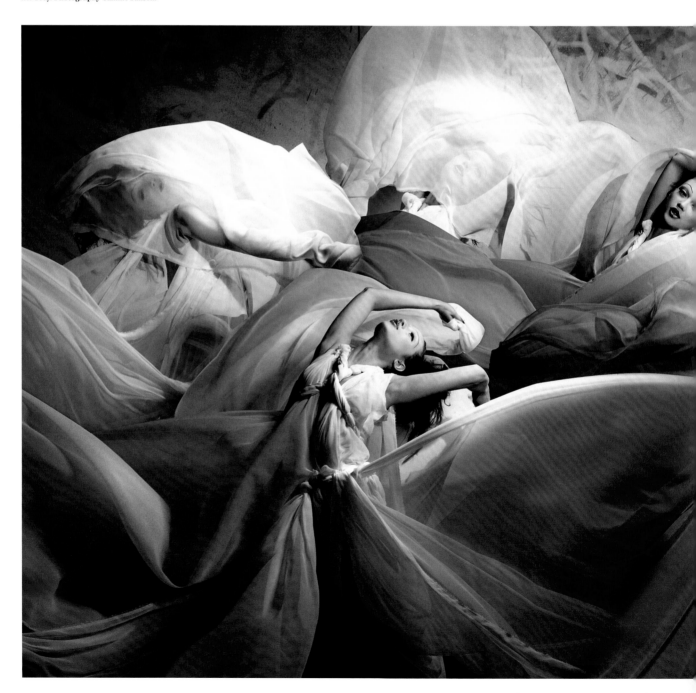

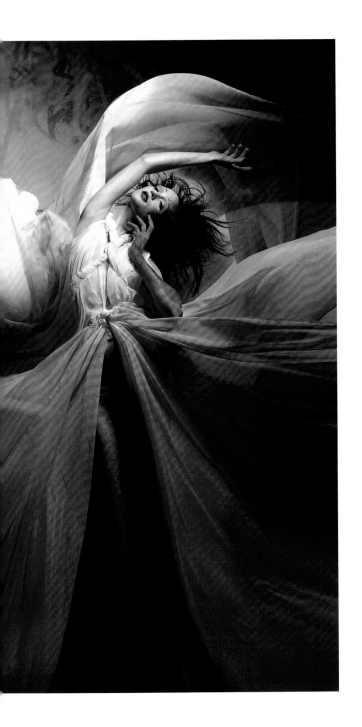

photographers and my portfolio just got better. I worked with all kinds of clients, no job was too small for me, and I often did unpaid work, believing it was a learning tool. Every job I did seemed to ead to another, and before I knew it I was working regularly and only doing test shoots for fun to improve my portfolio.

My big break

A chance meeting with another makeup artist led me to pitch for a job that was bigger than I had ever imagined. With our ideas and sketches we sealed the deal. It was to design for L'Oréal's 50th anniversary show with renowned hairdresser Trevor Sorbie. This was the beginning of my show work, which developed further and led to many more jobs, working with some of the best names in session hair. It gave me the confidence to work with regular teams on key London Fashion Week shows, both on-schedule and off-schedule.

As time passed I began to feel that I should start making some more decisive career choices as I already felt like a late starter, so I took the decision to start directing my portfolio – developing my own ideas, which had been whirling around in my brain for a long time. I teamed up with the photographer Camille Sanson, and this was the beginning of a new chapter of my life. No longer was I trying hard just to show off the makeup I could do, but also to art-direct timeless and beautiful imagery.

Making my mark

After seven years of working non-stop I took a deep breath and realized how far I had come. Working full time for retail, fashion shoots, and weddings, it suddenly dawned on me that there was a lot more to achieve. Developing my collaborations gave me hope that my work had a voice and that, together with a great team, I could achieve beautiful art work. As time passed I remember getting advice from a very

'Love, I believe, is the backbone of my success, and my inspiration. Everything else in life is a bonus.'

important PR person: 'You may be one of the best technical artists I have seen, but without celebrities or PR you are a needle in the haystack; come back when you have achieved this.' So that year I started to step outside the box and become a social artist, networking and putting feelers out to clients. Luckily I met celebrity stylist Karl Willett, with whom I had a lot in common; we share the same vision to create inherently thought-provoking and beautiful images. One collaboration led to another, he introduced me to some of his celebrity clients, and a new journey began. Working with beautiful celebrities widened the scope of my work and opened my eyes to another side of makeup, which is unspoken and private. You have to understand a client's needs and privacy, yet still work to the best of your creative ability at all times. This is one of the most challenging and rewarding aspects of my career now.

What makeup means to me

The meaning of makeup has never changed in my eyes. I believe that if you look good then you feel good! When you are happy with yourself it makes you smile. As a teenager battling with problem skin, my makeup was my sanctuary and gave me confidence. Just like any teenage girl systematically trying out a different makeup look every Friday! Makeup is fun, and confidence is beautiful. It's also all around us, from the reality of girls (and occasionally guys) walking down the street, to the fantasy of glossy magazines, theatre shows, TV series and films – makeup is an essential ingredient in everyday living. I am so thankful to be able to express my art in the form of makeup and hope you will enjoy reading this book, and ultimately be inspired to create, as I have.

Using makeup by The Makeup Store, commissioned for a music-themed issue of *M* magazine. **Photography** Camille Sanson.

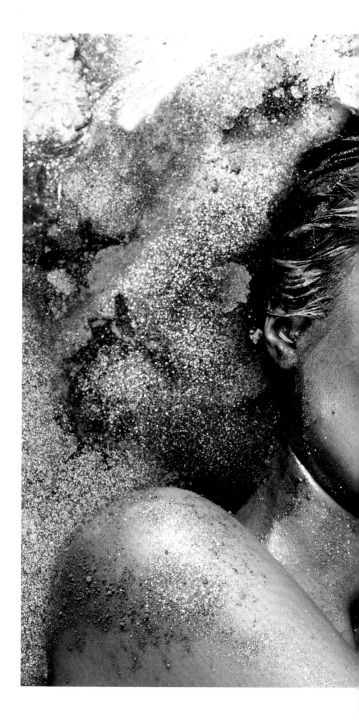

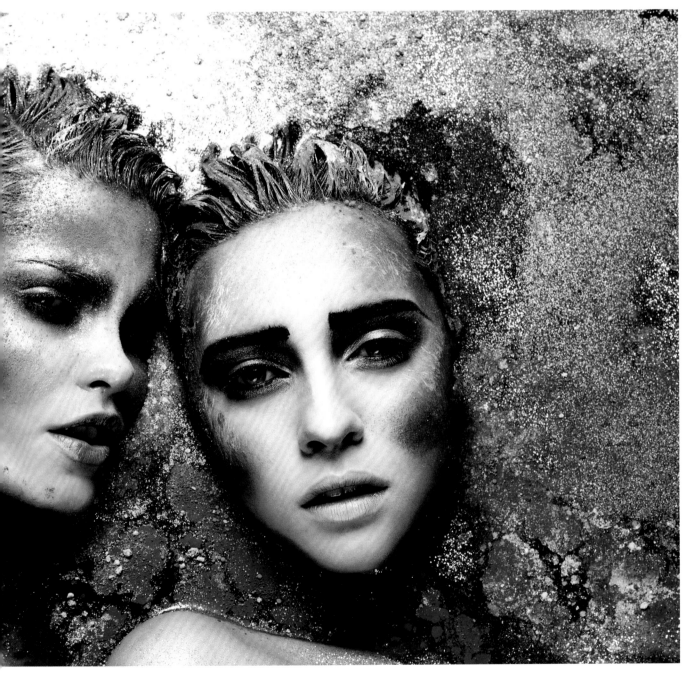

The A

of Be

Art

auty

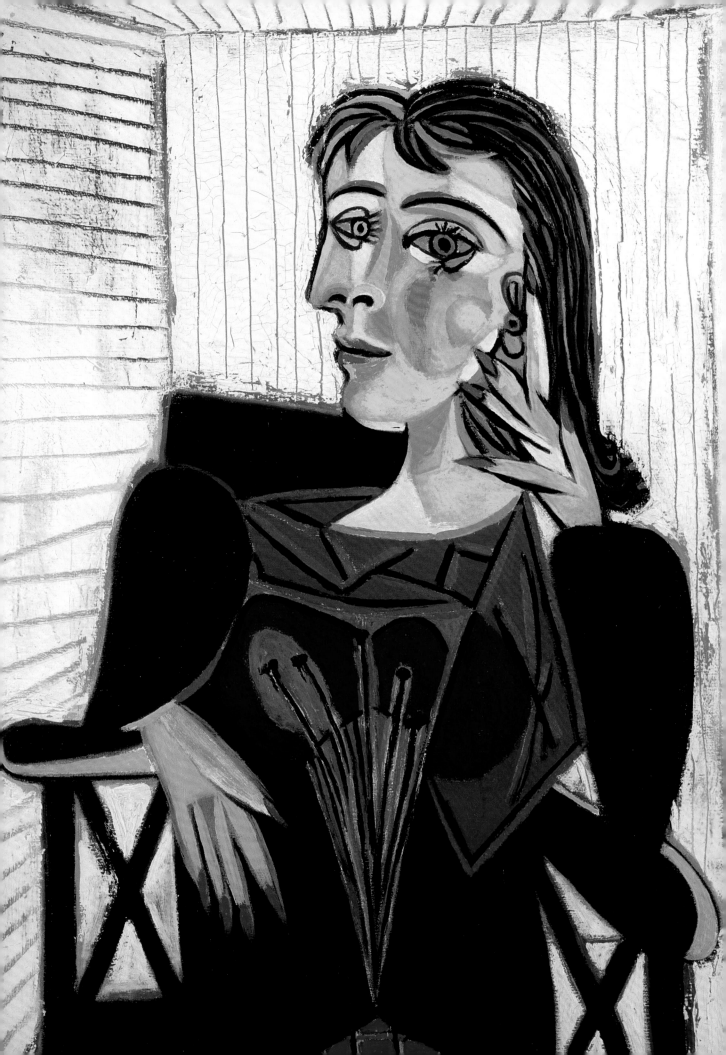

1. The Painters

Baroque, Impressionism, Cubism, Modernism, Pop Art, Expressionism

---

'*As with paintings, my aim is to create an emotional connection. All of us have an understanding of art inside us. Let your imagination go on a journey.*'

Pablo Picasso, Portrait de Dora Maar. 1937, Oil on canvas 92 x 65cm, Musee Picasso, Paris. © 2014 DACS

Opposite **Makeup** MAC Paint Pots (Groundwork, Constructivist), Eye Shadow (Bronze); Daniel Sandler Sculpt and Slim **Photography** Camille Sanson **Hair** Diana Moar using Bumble and Bumble **Styling** Karl Willett **Hats/Jewellery** Sorapol **Models** Joy, Gemma, Zoe Banks **Makeup Assistant** Loan Nguyen **Photography Assistant** Indigo Rohrer **Styling Assistant** Adele Pentland

'*Without atmosphere a painting is nothing.*'

– Rembrandt van Rijn (1606-1669)

Baroque

Portraits by the Baroque Dutch painter and etcher Rembrandt have all the allure of a deep and mysterious diamond mine. Dark caverns that sparkle here and there with shimmering touches of light – a technique known as 'chiaroscuro' from the Italian, *chiaro* meaning 'clear, light,' and *oscuro*, meaning 'obscure, dark'. The deft juxtaposition of the two and the gradual switch of one colour to the other gives a delicate, expressive image. As a young artist myself, this was one of the skills I tried to practise over and over again, studying most of Rembrandt's art for this lighting technique and bringing it into my own work. I love how the light draws you on a journey into the paintings like a spotlight.

Rembrandt was known for his limited palette, inspiring centuries of artists. Edvard Munch commented, 'In common with Michelangelo and Rembrandt I am more interested in the line, its rise and fall, than in colour.' In the final image, I mirrored this restrained use of brown tones and saturated colours for depth, diluted and blended for gradient, with pure white to highlight.

My model is sculpted and contoured using this effect, and with light and hard, dark brush strokes to achieve intensity and contrast. Like Rembrandt's portraits I have highlighted the nose in the direction of light, while the other tones are dramatized to give channels of depth between the floods of light. Understanding Rembrandt's work is one of the most important skills in makeup art that I have learnt.

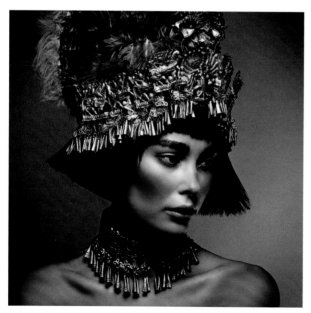
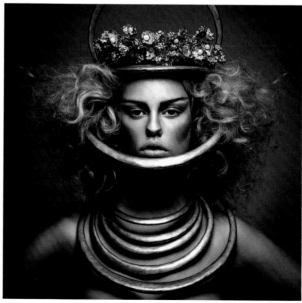

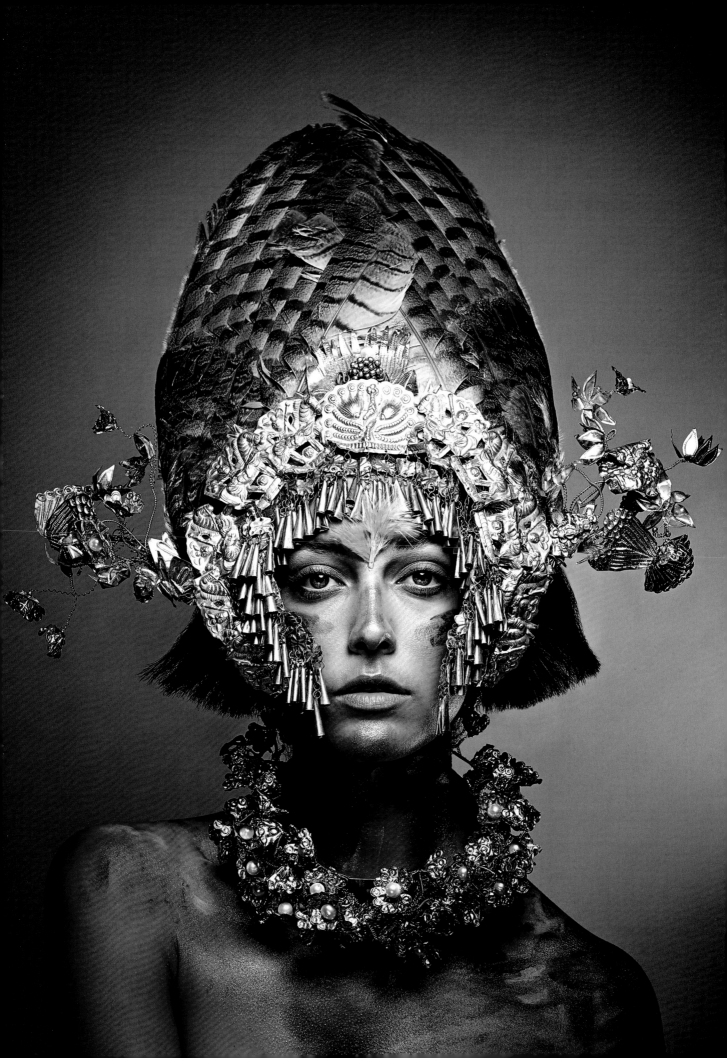

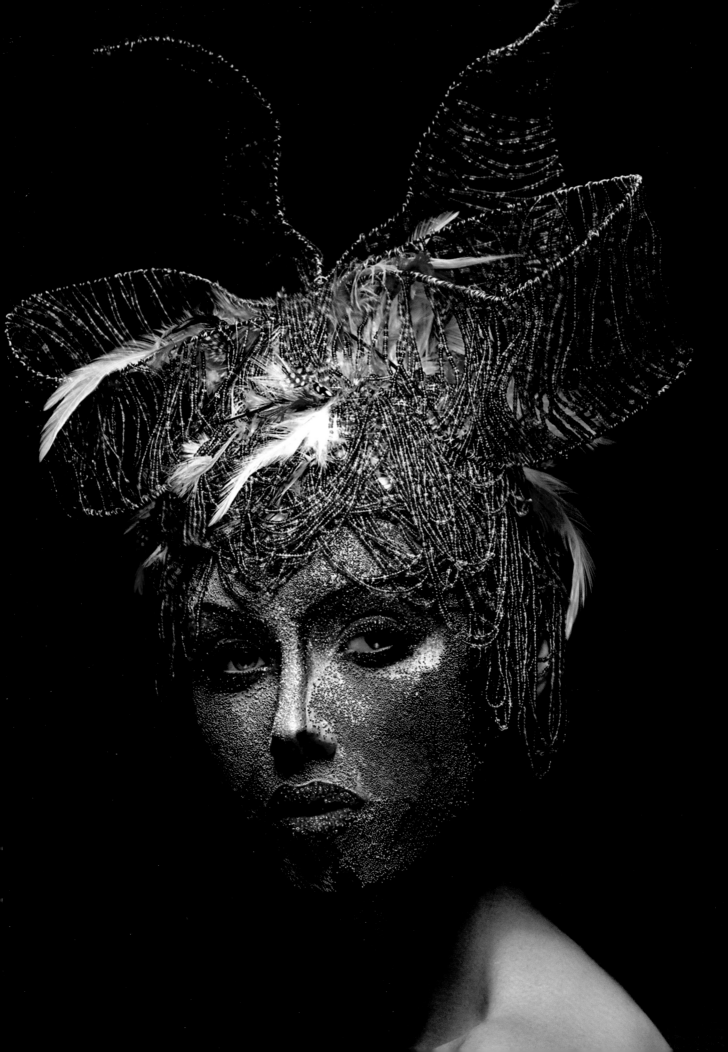

'*Colour is my day-long obsession, joy and torment.*'

– Claude Monet (1840-1926)

Impressionism

It's hard to believe now, but when Claude Monet first moved away from a classical painting style and began to exhibit his groundbreaking modern works alongside contemporaries Edgar Degas, Édouard Manet, Camille Pissarro and Pierre-Auguste Renoir in 1874, the show attracted widespread contempt. His 1872 work *Impression, Sunrise* was particularly scorned for its unfinished quality and wild, urgent brushstrokes. Furthermore, leaving parts of the raw canvas still visible was a revolutionary concept in nineteenth-century Paris. Revelling in their difference, the artists took the name 'Impressionists' after Monet's painting, and they sought to capture fleeting moments of everyday life, focusing on the play of light and the passing of the seasons.

A very important part of Impressionist art was understanding the effects of light on the colour of objects, and how colours blend into each other. In makeup this is just one of the ways I adapt my skills – working with light, texture and paint to enhance the beauty of the model.

Throwing aside convention, Monet often painted the same subject matter every day (in the 1910s and 1920s he almost exclusively painted the water lilies in his pond at Giverny), painting at different hours of the day and cropping so that only a portion of the view was seen.

In the finished image my aim was to capture this movement and to highlight areas to control the light on the model's skin. Beads and pigment are placed on top of my canvas; I let them sit where they want to, creating a free and unpredictable result. In the same way that Monet's famous bridge over the lily pond added structure to his unruly strokes, the headpiece in the photograph helps focus the eye while complementing the colours and textures. But as Monet himself rued, 'I'm not performing miracles, I'm using up and wasting a lot of paint.'

Makeup Kyrolan Supracolor Shimmering Vision Palette, Supracolor Interferenz Palette; Ciaté beads **Photography** Camille Sanson **Headpiece** Justin Smith **Model** Leila @ Profile

'One may have a blazing hearth in one's soul and yet no one ever came to sit by it. Passers-by see only a wisp of smoke from the chimney and continue on their way.'

– Vincent van Gogh (1853-1890)

At an early age I wanted to be an artist like Van Gogh. One of the saddest parts of his story is that he only became famous after his death. Much has been written about the great Dutch painter, his descent into mental illness and tragic suicide at the age of just 37. And it was this darkness that fuelled his creativity. Van Gogh embraced the style of the Impressionists after his move to Paris in 1886, and along with others developed the style into what became known as Post-Impressionism – further distorting form for expressive effect, and using unnatural colour from the realms of the imagination.

As with Monet's work, Van Gogh's technique was rhythmic and emotional – with strong content and form. The visible brushstrokes were infused with movement and surface tension. Bringing this poignancy to the image, I wanted to be light with brushstrokes and apply the texture of the beads freehand. I let them fall expressively to create an effect that's striking and powerful. Adding the headpiece, with its ripples of soft lace and black pearl-like embellishments, gives the image more depth and darkness, which further enhances the vivid colours.

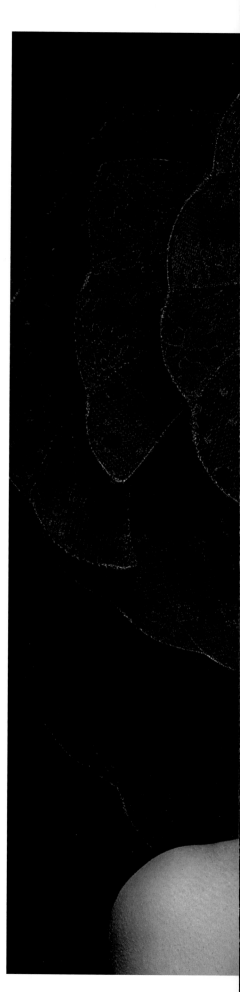

Makeup Kyrolan Supracolor Palette
24 Colors K, Eyelashes; Ciaté beads
Photography Camille Sanson **Hat** Justin
Smith **Model** Leila @ Profile

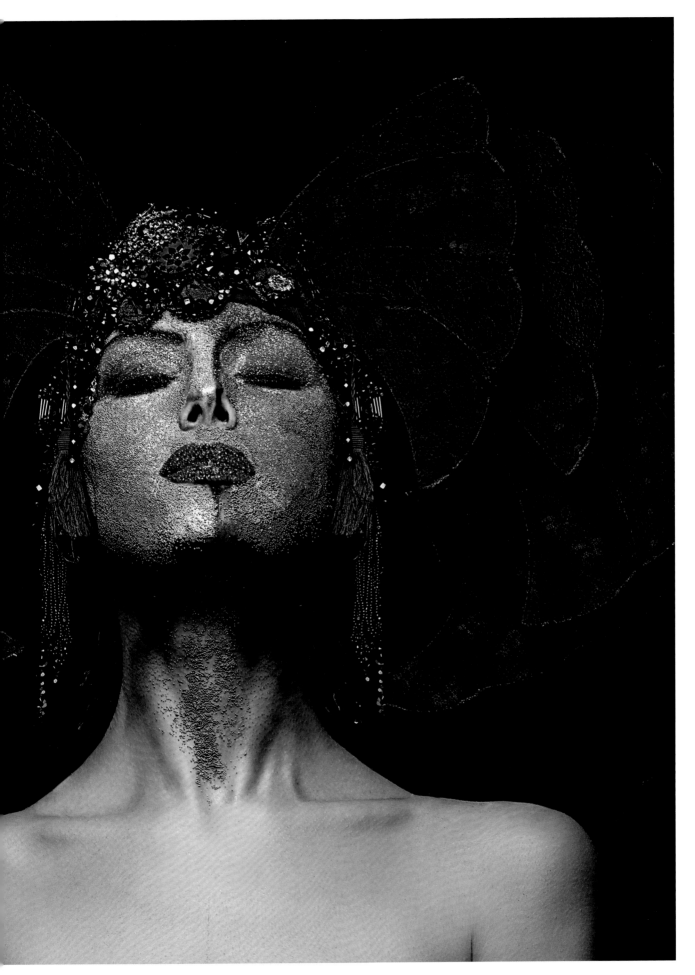

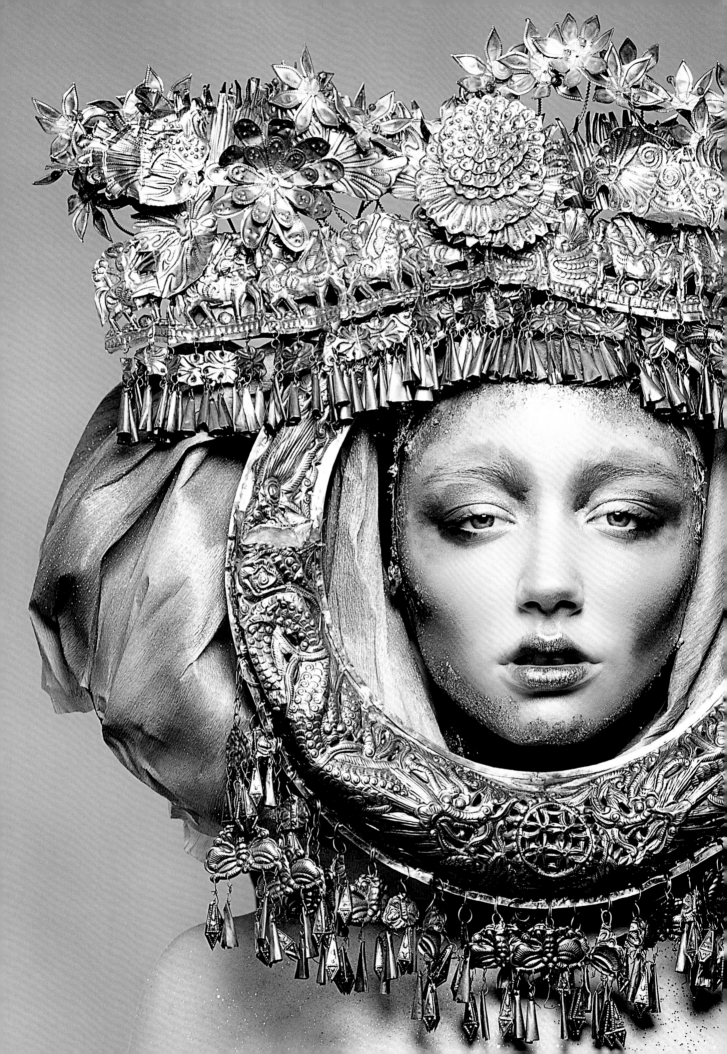

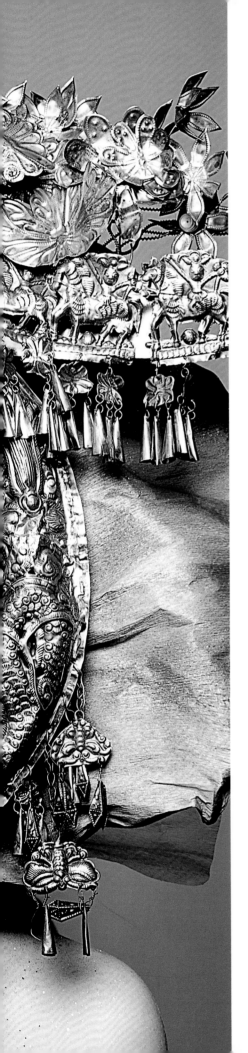

'Why shouldn't art be pretty? There are enough unpleasant things in the world.'

– Pierre-Auguste Renoir (1841–1919)

This shot was inspired by a French artist, Pierre-Auguste Renoir, who was a leading painter in the development of the Impressionist style. His paintings sparkled with light, and he used broken brushstrokes and bold combinations of pure complementary colours. Growing up studying the works of Renoir, I always noticed the strong celebration of beauty and feminine sensuality. The image seen here represents my freestyle method of painting, and a choice of colours that are saturated and vivid. The work of Renoir had movement, and through his light paintstrokes the figures and details of his scenes would fuse together with one another, and with their surroundings.

Makeup Kryolan Shimmering Event Foundation (Silver), Ultra Foundation TV White, Supracolor UV-Dayglow Shades Eye Shadow Palettes (Dubai, Dublin), Faceliner, Polyester Glimmer (Gold), UV-Dayglow Compact Color Palette, HD Cream Liner; gold leaf **Photography** Camille Sanson **Hair** Diana Moar **Styling** Karl Willett **Hat** Sorapol **Model** Claudia @ Premier

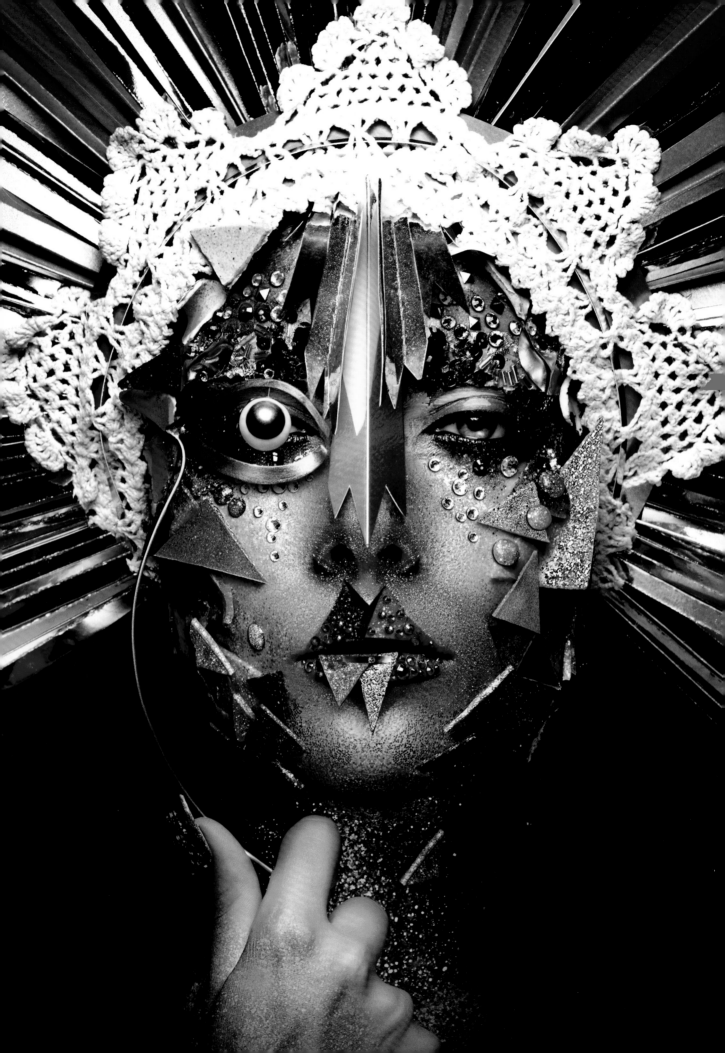

'*Why do two colours, put one next to the other, sing? Can one really explain this? No. Just as one can never learn how to paint.*'

– Pablo Picasso (1881–1973)

Cubism

There are as many sides to Pablo Picasso as there are angles in one of his Cubist masterpieces. The Spanish expatriate in Paris expressed himself as a painter, sculptor, printmaker, ceramicist, stage designer, poet and playwright. A man with burning passions for both his art and for women, he was a serial philanderer. Out of the seven most important women in his life, two killed themselves, two went mad, and one of his loves lay dying of tuberculosis while he carried on an affair with another woman. It was his opinion that 'There are only two types of women: goddesses and doormats.'

But it was his fiery Iberian sensibilities that also set canvases ablaze with colour. Picasso is one of my favourite painters because of his use of colour and his balance between harmony and complete chaos. My interpretation and inspiration came from one of his greatest works, *The Weeping Woman* (1937), which has an arresting intensity, edges jagged with grief. The subject of the painting is Dora Maar, Picasso's lover and private muse. The educated and political Maar was the rival of his mistress Marie-Thérèse Walter, who had a daughter with the artist, named Maya. Maar herself was infertile, and Picasso often painted her torment. I wanted to achieve that sense of beauty and sadness that draws you to look through her eyes and tell a story. As Picasso said, 'Good artists copy; great artists steal.'

Makeup Kryolan Supracolor Shimmering Vision Palette, Supracolor Interferenz Palette, Polyester Glimmer (Gold, Light Gold), Red Gelatin, HD Cream Liner (Aqua), Kajal Pencil (Black); Swarovski Crystals **Photography** Camille Sanson **Hair** Diana Moar **Styling** Karl Willett **Eyepiece** Vicki Sarge **Hat** Ivana Nohel **Model** Zoe Banks **Makeup Assistants** Kelly Mendiola and Lolo Page **Styling Assistant** Adele Pentland **Nails** The Freelance Workspace using VuDu Nails. Special thanks to Hannah Maestranzi

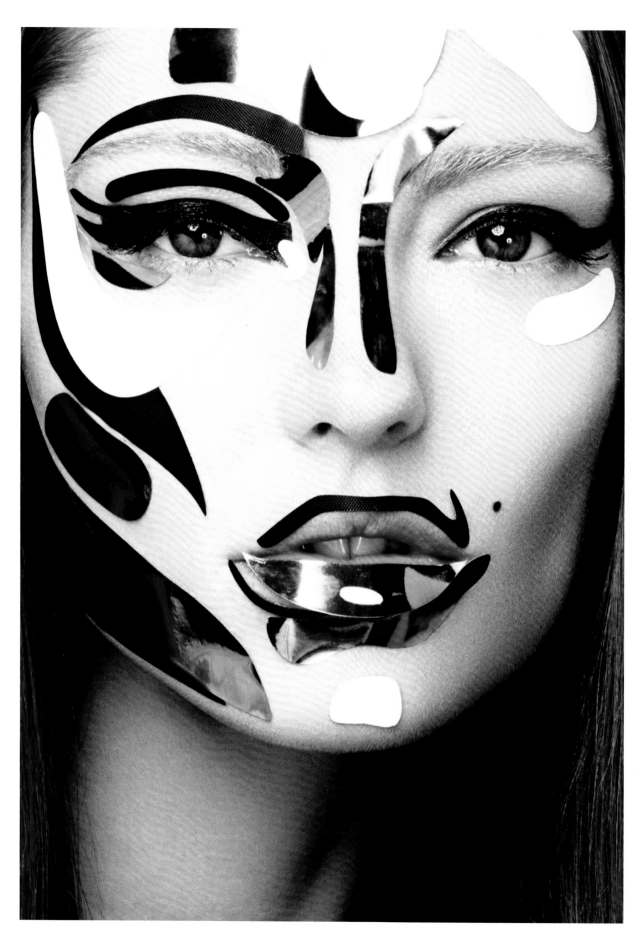

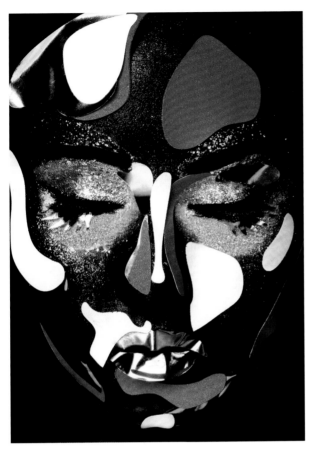

Opposite **Makeup** MAC Face and
Body Foundation (White), Fluidline
(Blacktrack); Face•Lace **Photography** Mark
Cant **Model** Ellie

Left **Makeup** MAC Paintsticks, Glitter
(Crystallized Lime, Turquoise, 3D Brass Gold,
3D Silver), Mixing Medium; Face•Lace
Photography Catherine Harbour **Model** Rae
Matthews @ Nevs

Using Face•Lace to create the look

I collaborated with Phyllis Cohen, makeup artist
and inventor of Face•Lace, to produce these images.
Here she explains how she created the custom-made
face appliqués that I used to create the looks on these
and other pages in this book.

'When I met with Lan to discuss how we might
collaborate she expressed a desire to use Face•Lace
to create a Pop-art typeface using blocks of colour.
Immediately the wheels of my imagination started
to spin … I saw faces mapped like geographic,
topographic diagrams, with the planes of the face
separated into shapes. Before I began as a makeup
artist I had extensive training as an illustrator.
I had a brilliant tutor who taught us portraiture by
teaching us the planes of the face. This was a system
he devised which broke the facial structure down
into about 40 shapes, which we had to memorize and
use when sketching from life.

When I came to create these maps for the Face•Lace
blocks for Lan, I researched interesting uses of colour
on painted faces. I studied in particular the paintings
of Alexej von Jawlensky, the first artist that popped
in my head when Lan said she wanted something
like a cross between Warhol and Cubism. Jawlensky
used flat blocks of bold colour for his portraits. I

realized that in order to translate this concept of
blocks of colour into Face•Lace, I had to make a
study of a face in a light that accentuated the planes
of bone structure. I pulled out my favourite books
of Hollywood portraits. I enlarged to life-size a
straight-on portrait of a young Joan Crawford shot
by George Hurrell – one of the great Hollywood
photographers.

Using this printout I carefully copied all of the
highlights, mid-tones and shadows on her face.
I worked out that I could represent the deepest
shadows in black, and the lightest highlights in white.
The mid-tones could be represented in any mid-tone
colour. In the end I did all the mid-tone shapes,
about 20 altogether, in seven sets of colours, both
matt and metallic.

I figured that the playful and interchanging use of
different colours and textures for the mid-tone shapes
is what would give the final look of the Pop-art face
its expressiveness. This is what I noticed from the
artistic references I collected – that the mid-tones
of the portrait could be a bold mix of bright colours
and work brilliantly to describe the face, as long as
the darkest shadows and lightest highlights were
anchored in exactly the right place.'

'Colour is all. When colour is right, form is right. Colour is everything, colour is vibration like music; everything is vibration.'

– Marc Chagall (1887–1985)

Modernism

The pioneering Modernist Marc Chagall worked prolifically in a diverse range of mediums, including painting, book illustrations, stained glass, stage sets, ceramic, tapestries and fine art prints. In another dimension perhaps he would have traded his tubes of oil for a wheelie bag full of face powders and pigments. Pablo Picasso commented in the 1950s that after the death of Matisse, 'Chagall will be the only painter left who understands what colour really is.' His vibrant, swirling gem tones of cobalt, ruby and jasper, and evocative, otherworldly figures leap off the canvas.

More than simply a colour palette muse, Chagall's real genius was in creating a world where anything was possible – flying horses, green donkeys, man embracing his animalistic side – a recurring theme of his work is his fantastical man/beast hybrids. I was drawn to his dreamlike ideas, and his mixing of a new style of modern art with Eastern European Jewish folk culture.

Picasso said that he was not crazy about Chagall's 'flying violins and all the folklore, but his canvases are really painted, not just thrown together.' He added: 'There's never been anybody since Renoir who has the feeling for light that Chagall has.' So what can we take from this? A sense of exuberance – and, from a technical perspective, that we can balance blocks of wash colour with clearly defined edges to give a modernist, graphic effect. We can also channel the artist's sensibility for romantic beauty, as shown by his oft-painted scenes of lovers. Though Chagall lived for years under the oppressive grey skies of Vitebsk in modern-day Belarus, he infused his day-to-day scenes with vibrant hues.

To create my image I was inspired by a hat designed by J. Smith Esquire; it had the key elements of vibrant colour and graphic shapes. I loved the fact that when in place it sat like a stained-glass window, framing the face, and the delicacy of its construction could be fully appreciated. To complement the look I brought out the model's eyes and darkened other areas to keep the intensity of depth. The play between shadow and light maintains the mystery.

Makeup Kyrolan Supracolor Palette 24 Colors K **Photography** Camille Sanson **Hat** Justin Smith **Model** Leila @ Profile

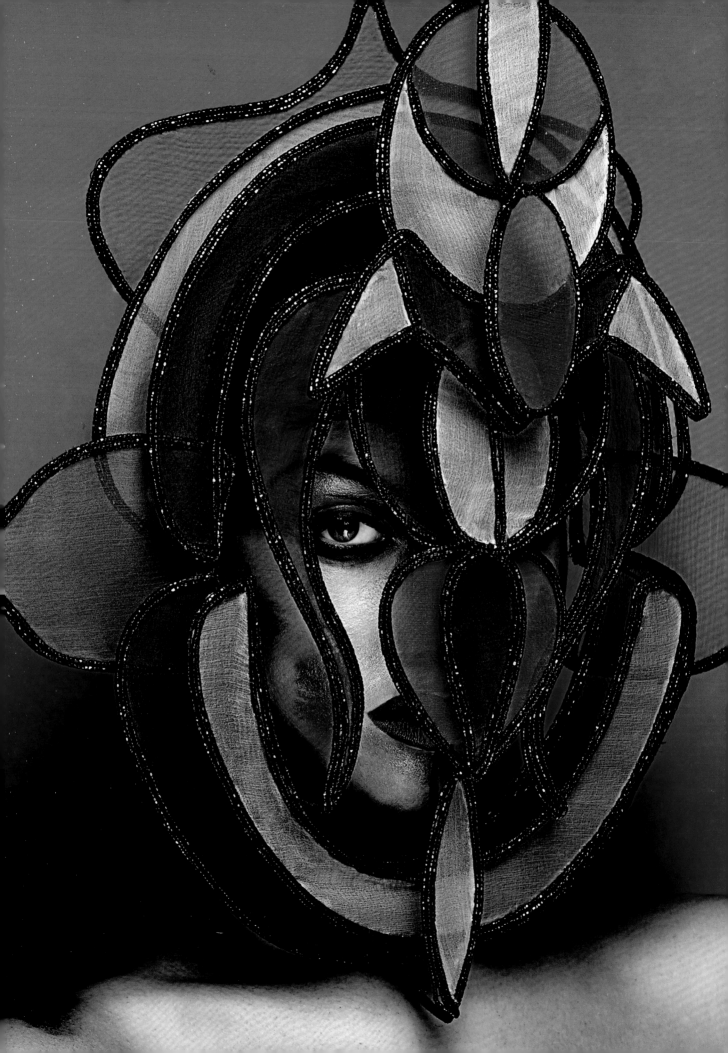

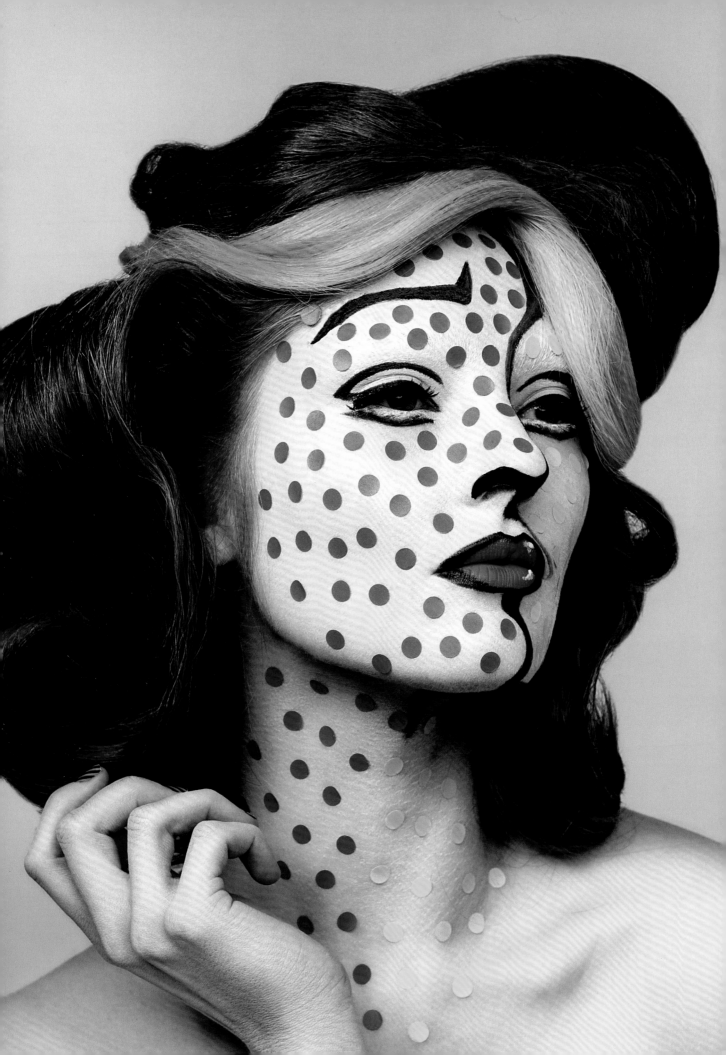

'Art doesn't transform. It just plain forms.'

– Roy Lichtenstein (1923–1997)

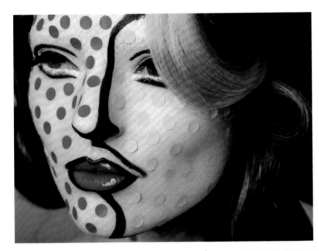

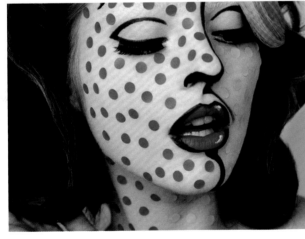

Pop art

Pop art originated in Britain in the mid-1950s, and found its spiritual home in late 1950s/1960s' consumer culture. The genre turned conventional ideas of art on their head, repackaging commonplace motifs from the worlds of advertising, celebrity and news for a gluttonous second helping by the viewing public. Rather than a defining style or medium, Pop art was typified by its irreverent, devil-may-care attitude. 'I'm not really sure what social message my art carries, if any. And I don't really want it to carry one,' explained Lichtenstein. 'I'm not interested in the subject matter to try to teach society anything, or to try to better our world in any way.'

The images on these pages are my interpretation of Lichtenstein's copy of a panel by the famous American comic book artist Jack Kirby, hich is very much in the spirit of Pop art. I wanted to recreate his popular cartoon-like images using bold colours to give that 'POW!' feeling. Playing with primary colours, and keeping the lines and signature Ben-Day dots very simple, I worked with the face and contours to ensure the look was still beautiful and balanced. Adding false lashes, and bringing out the lines of contour around the eyes – combined with the model's kitsch expression – gave the image an exaggerated femininity.

Makeup Kryolan TV Paint Stick (TV White), Supracolor Palette 24 Colors K, HD Cream Liner (Ebony), Eylure Volume lashes **Photography** Catherine Harbour **Hair** Chie Sato using Label.m **Model** Ellie **Makeup Assistants** Yuko Fredriksson, Kelly Mendiola and Eoin Whelan

'Everybody must have a fantasy.'

– Andy Warhol (1928–1987)

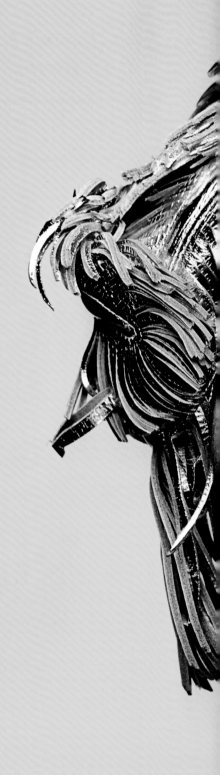

Long before Facebook, Twitter and Instagram there was the ultimate social networker – Andy Warhol – who moved seamlessly between the worlds of fashion, music, art and film.

After moving to New York he became a successful commercial illustrator, with a client roster that included Columbia Records, *Glamour, Harper's Bazaar*, NBC, Tiffany & Co. and *Vogue*. By the 1950s he was exhibiting as an artist in his own right, and throughout his life his work encompassed many media, including drawing, painting, printmaking, photography, silk screening and sculpture.

A neurological disorder in his youth left Warhol shut indoors, poring over celebrity magazines and DC comics, and it was themes of publicity and caricature that continued to attract him as an adult.

The look I have created here was inspired by the iconic 1962 silkscreen painting *Marilyn Diptych*. I have always been fascinated by Warhol's cartoon-like images and particularly loved his Marilyn Monroe paintings. Often his work was quite comical and had no explanation. The artist himself said at the time, 'Art is what you can get away with.' Using basic techniques with paint and makeup I tried to capture the humour of my model and take her to that place of Pop art.

Makeup Kryolan HD Cream Liner in Ebony, HD Micro Foundation Cream Palette and Colors MFC1 **Photography** Camille Sanson **Hat** Justin Smith **Model** Leila @ Profile

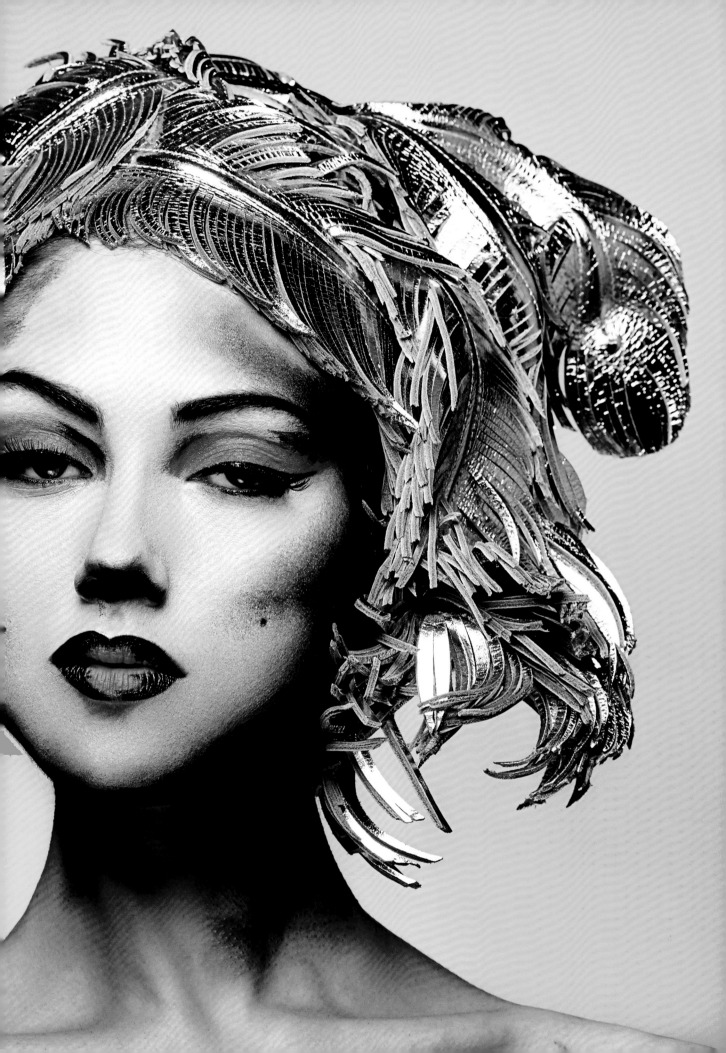

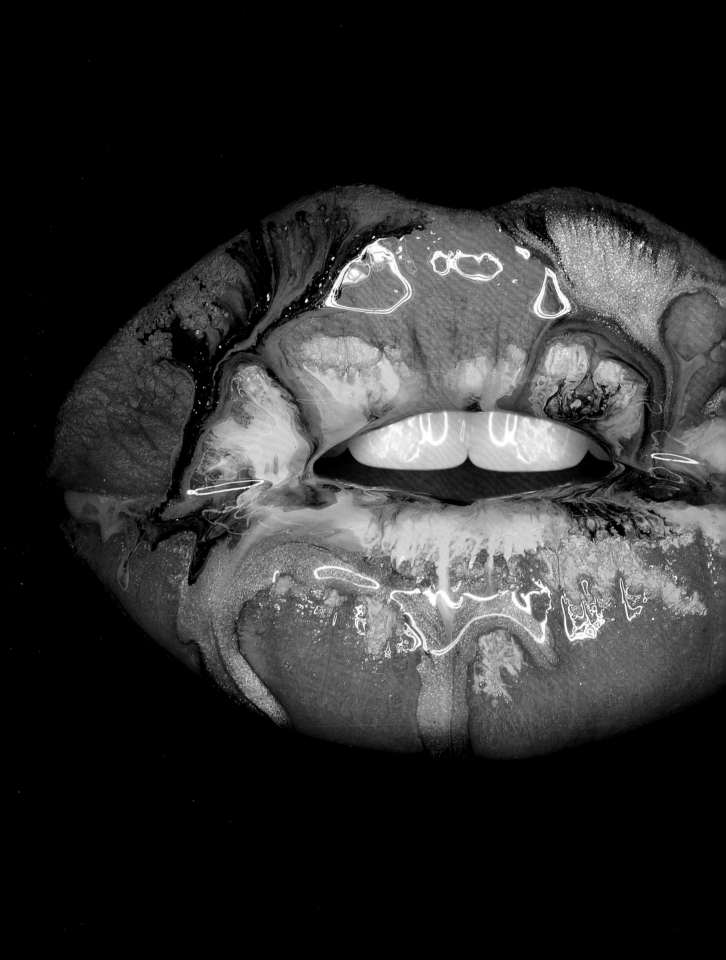

'When I am painting I have a general notion as to what I am about. I can control the flow of paint: there is no accident.'

– Jackson Pollock (1912-1956)

Expressionism

A major painter in abstract art and expressionism, Jackson Pollock was known for his unique style of drip painting. I tried to reference his style with fluid paint that started at a point and explored with moving it to create a fluid trail. Working on lips was tricky due to the force of gravity, so I had to figure out how to slow the process down. Laying a gloss mixture underneath it made the paint thicker and slower to move.

Layering all the different colours at different points gave a unique colour mixture, and movement that was interesting to watch. Applying it with a brush at different angles also affected the movement and colour balance. Working this way I became so completely engrossed that I forgot what I was doing; it became an instinct to just keep adding and taking away constantly. It takes on a life of its own and you only see how beautiful the results are when you walk away and see it captured in a picture. The colours were all accidental and the mixtures gave a different image every second.

Makeup; Kryolan High Gloss, Lip Stain; MAC Lipsticks (Ruby Woo, Lady Danger), Lipglass; Obsessive Compulsive Cosmetics Lip Tar
Photography John Oakley **Model** Micheala

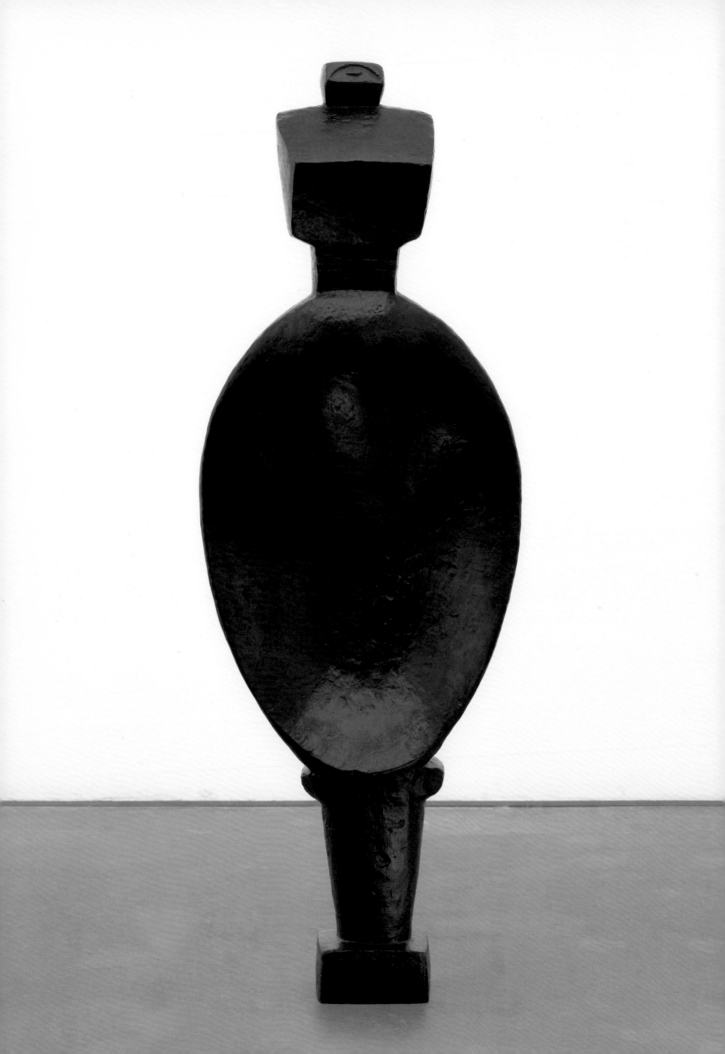

2. The Sculptors

Alberto Giacometti, Anish Kapoor, Henry Moore, Damien Hirst

'*Working with texture and three dimensions through freedom of materials and process brings the human form to life and evokes deeper feelings.*'

Alberto Giacometti, Spoon
Woman, 1927 (1953 version)
(plaster), 146.5x51.6x21.5cm.
Collection Fondation Alberto
& Annette Giacometti.

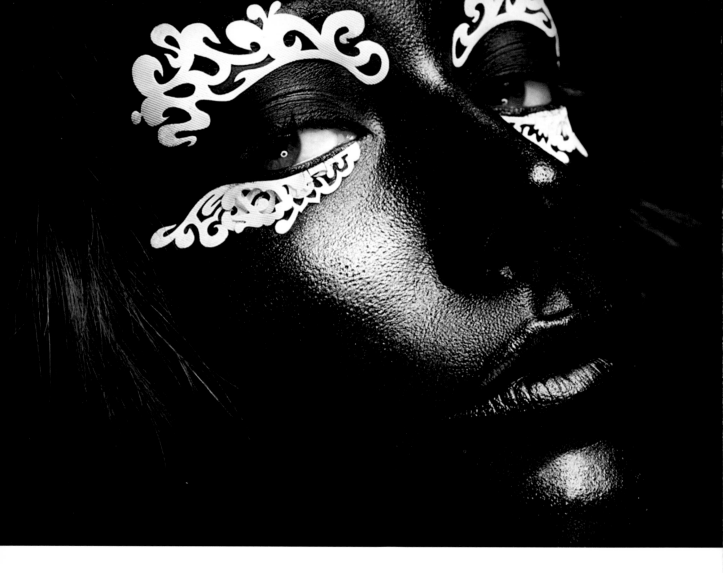

Alberto Giacometti

Giacometti's key obsession as an artist was to capture the essence of a person. Studying his portrait subject for an age (he once made his friend James Lord sit for 18 days straight), he would repeatedly carve away until the sculpted figure was eroded at its edges, with rough texture, the face and body deconstructed, face right down to the nails. The sculptures are unique and haunting representations of the human form. The figures are generally stretched and elongated like a ghostly shadow. The artist himself once said that he was sculpting not the human figure but 'the shadow that is cast.'

I often wonder what he would have been feeling at the time he was making the pieces. Giacometti's work has a feeling of isolation that is part of his unique style. He was always a favourite of mine while studying art. In the latter part of his career, he moved away from surrealism and favoured existentialism – searching for meaning in a seemingly absurd world.

Famously Giacometti would continue to revisit old works. 'That's the terrible thing: the more one works on a picture, the more impossible it becomes to finish it,' he admitted. I took this as inspiration and reworked some of my old techniques to create these looks. I let the outcome of the final image be influenced by how I was feeling at the time, letting the clothes and hats I used influence what I was going to create with the makeup.

Makeup Kryolan Supracolor Greasepaint in Black; Face•Lace **Photography** Camille Sanson **Styling** Karl Willett **Jacket and Skirt** Ivan Pilja **Hat** Victoria Grant **Model** Zoe Banks @ MOT Models **Makeup Assistants** Kelly Mendiola and Lolo Page **Photography Assistant** Indigo Rohrer **Nails** The Freelance Workspace using VuDu Nails

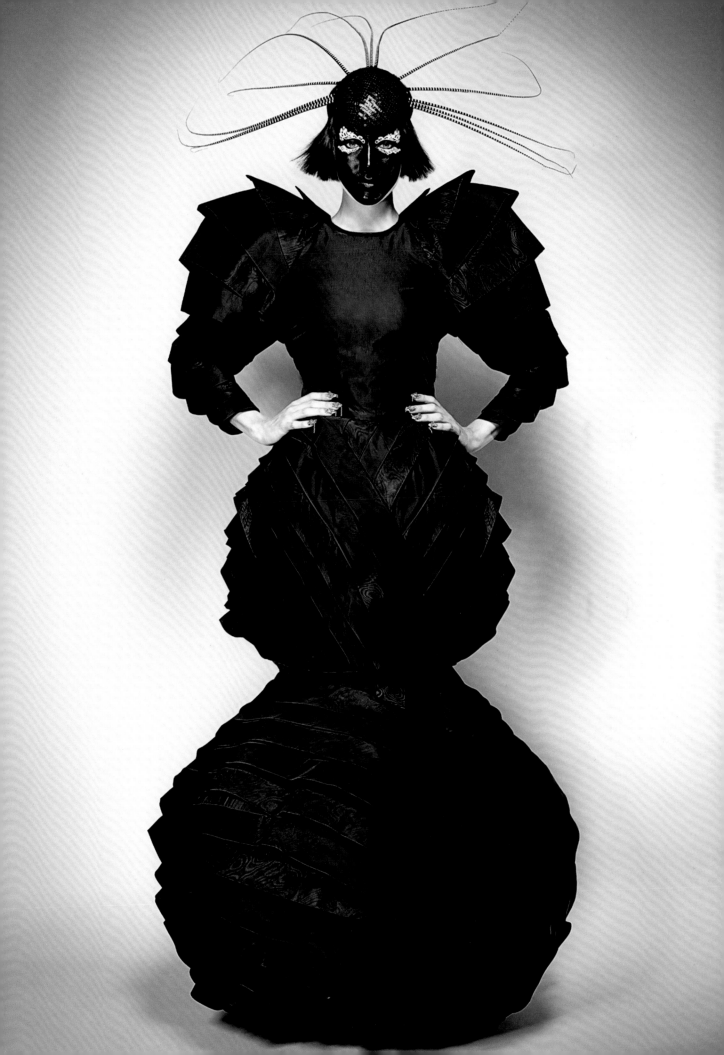

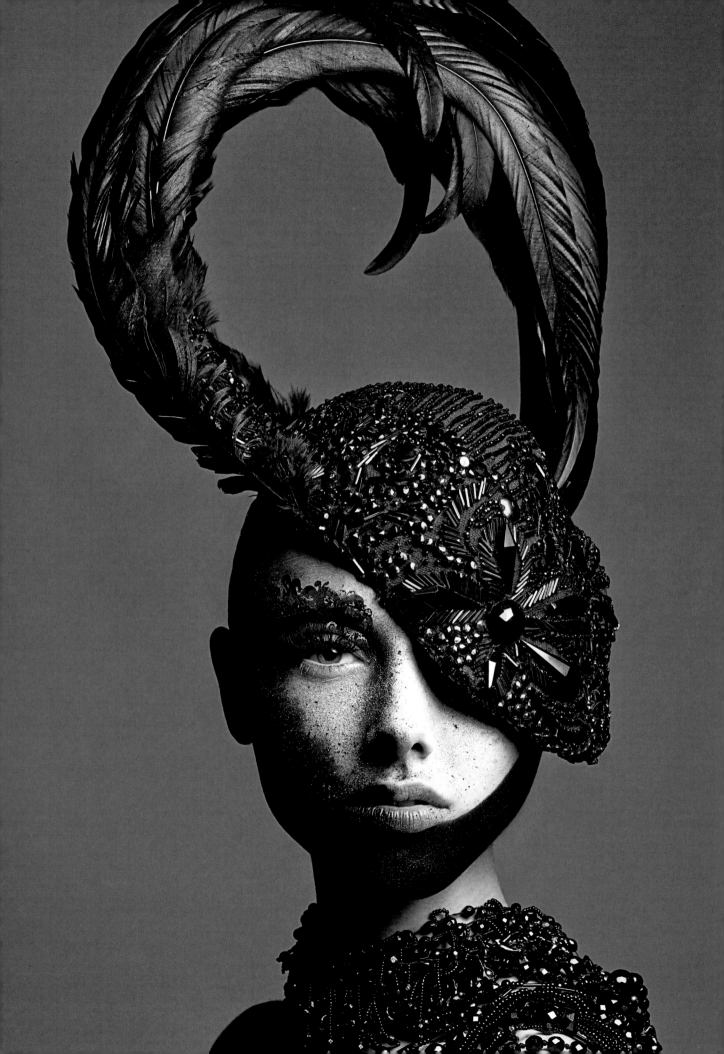

'*The human face is as strange to me as a countenance, which, the more one looks at it, the more it closes itself off and escapes by the steps of unknown stairways.*'

– Alberto Giacometti (1901–1966)

Makeup MAC Full Coverage Foundation
(White), Greasepaint Stick (Black), Pigment
(Dark Soul); Face•Lace; Paperself eyelashes
Photography Camille Sanson **Headpiece**
Justin Smith **Model** Leila @ Profile

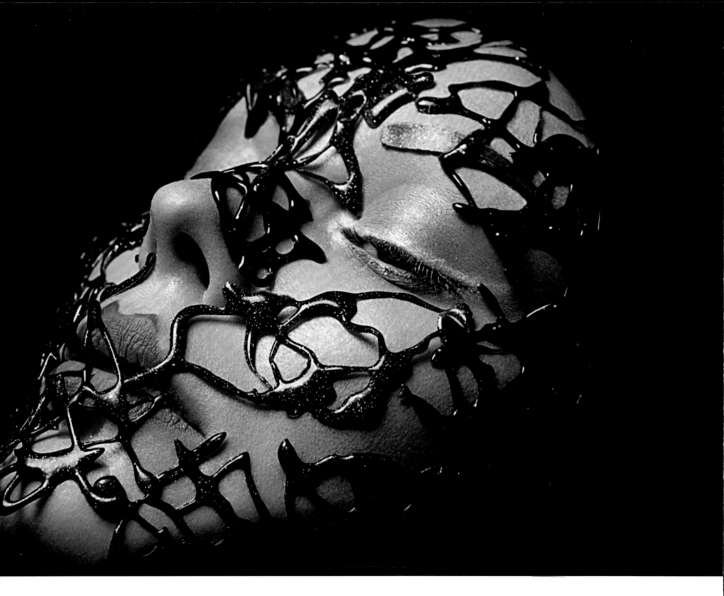

Working in three dimensions

Picasso, while most famous for his paintings, was a fan of the plastic arts, working in mediums that could be moulded or modelled. Fittingly, it was the use of special-effects gelatin by makeup artist Hannah Maestranzi that gave the final image its three-dimensional makeup effect. Here she explains how to use this advanced technique.

What is gelatin and how does it work?

'Gelatin is a medium widely used for three-dimensional makeup. It is easy to apply and safe for the skin, and is often used in special-effects makeup to simulate skin anomalies such as severe burn injuries, scaring, pimples and boils. Gelatin is an excellent medium for prosthetic makeup due to its flesh-like consistency, elasticity, high tear threshold, and ability to capture fine detail when prepared in pre-made moulds.

'Gelatin can often be found under different brand names such as Kryolan Gelafix Skin, Mouldlife FX Nuggets or Glynn McKay Gelglyk. Gelatin can be bought as powder and mixed to the required consistency with water, glycerin and flocking – but it is generally used and sold in slabs, nuggets or even

in a pipette bottle for convenience. The colour of gelatin can also vary widely, from clear and flesh-toned to blood red.'

Heating

'Before starting to work with gelatin, it must always be heated. It can be heated in two ways, depending on whether the product is going to be used directly on skin, or put into a pre-made mould. If applying directly on to skin, it must be heated in a bain-marie so it won't overheat and become too hot for skin application. It's best to cut the gelatin into small cubes first so it melts quicker. As soon as it's melted, apply straight away, as once it starts to cool it will begin to solidify.

'If using a mould, it can be heated in the microwave. First cut it up into small cubes, then place in a plastic bowl and heat for a couple of seconds. Once viscous it can be painted/poured into a pre-made mould. The great thing about gelatin, especially when using it for the first time, is the ability to recycle it – so long as it isn't heated beyond a certain threshold – so if there are any mistakes or flaws it can be melted repeatedly.'

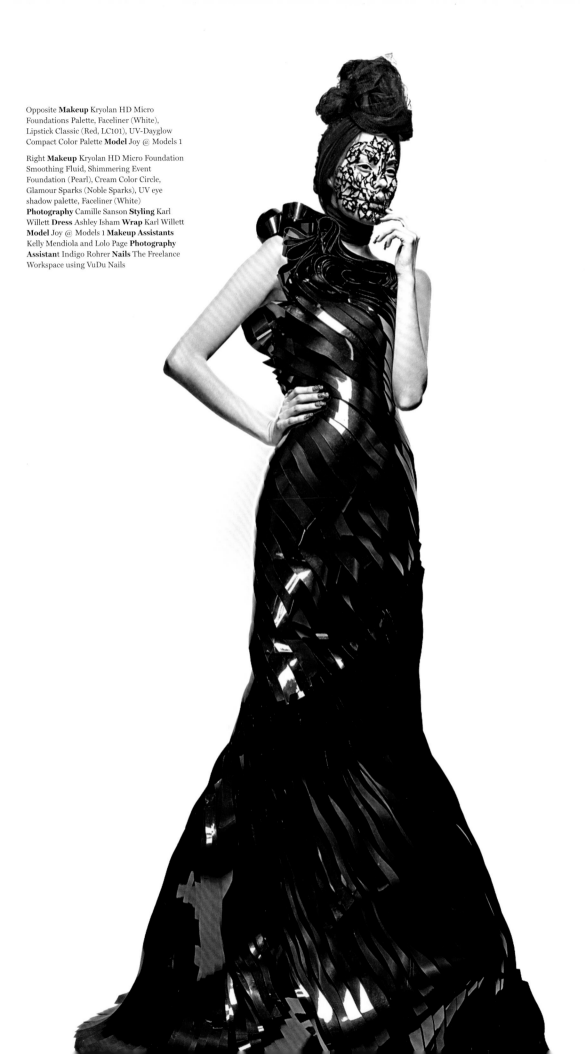

Opposite **Makeup** Kryolan HD Micro
Foundations Palette, Faceliner (White),
Lipstick Classic (Red, LC101), UV-Dayglow
Compact Color Palette **Model** Joy @ Models 1

Right **Makeup** Kryolan HD Micro Foundation
Smoothing Fluid, Shimmering Event
Foundation (Pearl), Cream Color Circle,
Glamour Sparks (Noble Sparks), UV eye
shadow palette, Faceliner (White)
Photography Camille Sanson **Styling** Karl
Willett **Dress** Ashley Isham **Wrap** Karl Willett
Model Joy @ Models 1 **Makeup Assistants**
Kelly Mendiola and Lolo Page **Photography
Assistant** Indigo Rohrer **Nails** The Freelance
Workspace using VuDu Nails

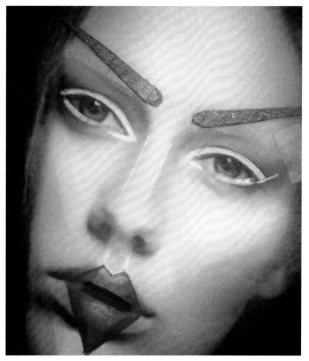
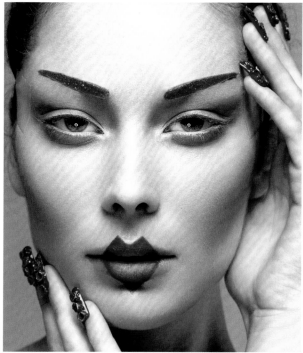

Colouring

'I cut the gelatin into small pieces, placed in a plastic bowl, and added a few drops of brightly coloured, water-based liquid makeup, neon green, blue, pink, white and black. Only a few drops of liquid makeup are needed to make the gelatin an opaque colour, as too much fluid can change the consistency of the gelatin, making it brittle. Once the coloured gelatin was melted I quickly added the glitter and stirred. If this colour batch solidified before I had finished using it I re-melted in the microwave. Please note that I was using polyester glitter, which is safe to use in a microwave.'

Throwing shapes

'We started with simple patterns that could be used to adorn the face for various looks, such as dots and triangles.

'The dots are the easiest to make; simply take the melted gelatin and using the end of a brush dot on to a clean flat surface – I used a steel mixing palette. This makes the gelatin cool and solidify almost instantly; it can then be peeled off and used to stick on to the face straight away.

'Other freehand shapes were the squiggles or the mini 'Gaudí-esque' shapes. Again, picking up some melted gelatin on the end of the brush I allowed the gelatin to fall and drip on to the flat surface in a random way, overlapping itself, creating a lace-like piece. As theses pieces were made freehand, every single one was unique.

'For shapes such as triangles or eyebrows, a mould had to be made using plasticine or modelling clay. The plasticine was rolled out as even and thin as possible on a clean, flat surface. I then carved out my shapes, such as a triangle, with a scalpel. The negative space was then filled with the gelatin, and, once dry, the shapes were peeled out. To create multiple copies of shapes with consistency a mould would usually be cast in plaster. To smooth any irregular edges I lightly brushed the shapes with a little witch hazel.'

Application

'To apply, Pros-Aide medical-grade adhesive was used. Please note the glue has to be dried completely before applying a gelatin piece. As gelatin is a non-porous material the glue will not dry properly, meaning pockets can develop and therefore leave the piece is more susceptible to peeling away.'

Above left and opposite Lan's 3D smudge charts.

Above right **Makeup** Kryolan HD Micro Foundations Palette, Faceliner (White), Lipstick Classic (Red, LC101), UV-Dayglow Compact Color Palette **Photography** Camille Sanson **Model** Joy @ Models 1 **Nails** The Freelance Workspace using VuDu Nails

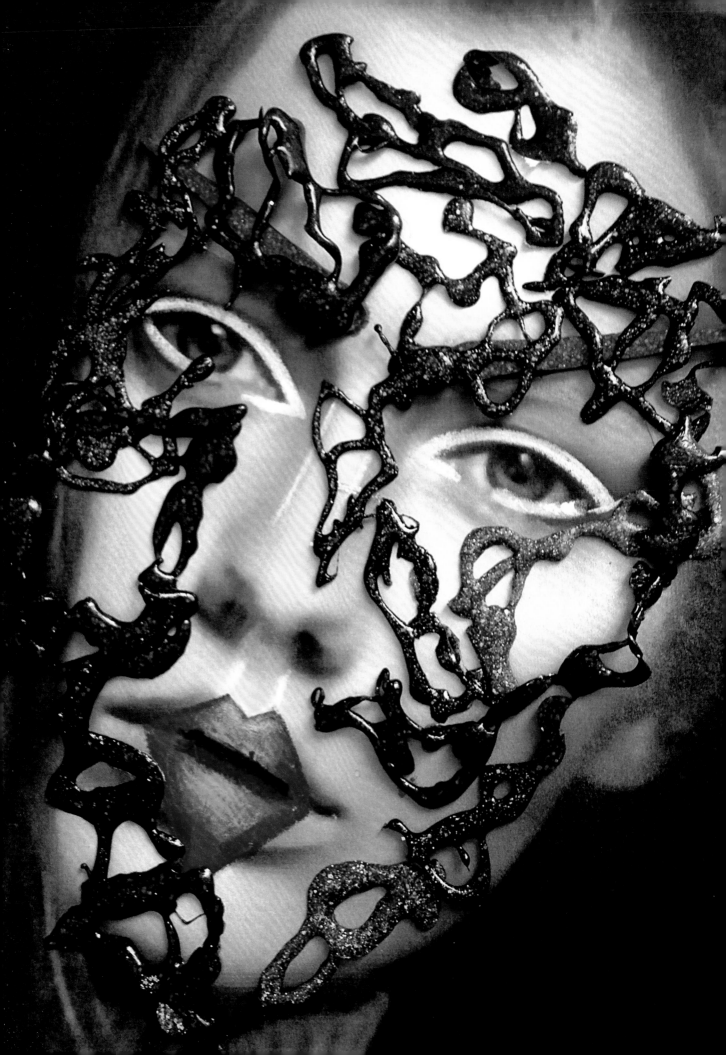

'Artists don't make objects. Artists make mythologies.'
– Anish Kapoor (b. 1954)

Anish Kapoor

Bombay-born London resident Anish Kapoor is one of the most decorated sculptors of our time – winning many awards, including the Turner Prize in 1991, and receiving the Unilever Commission for the Turbine Hall at Tate Modern in 2002. Despite their very physical materiality and construction in granite, limestone, marble, plastic and pigment, many of his vast geometric works recede into the distance or distort the space around them.

Kapoor's gargantuan public works grace cities across the globe, and it is his work with reflective surfaces – polished steel mirrors and water in a controlled environment – that inspired this image. The beautiful, smooth surfaces and giant sculptures by Kapoor take you on a physical journey of mind and body. And as Kapoor states, 'All ideas grow out of other ideas.' I have applied these concepts to the human form. The otherworldly images I have created on this and the following few pages are inspired by the sense of movement and colour, texture and reflections that dominate Kapoor's work.

Right **Makeup** Kryolan Supracolor Palette 24 Colors K, Aquacolor Liquid, UV Paint S12, 070, 509, 071, 510, R21, R27 032, 080, TK2, Glamour Sparks, Multi Gel Glitters (Silver, Lavender, Light Gold, Pearl White) **Photography** Camille Sanson **Hair** Jose Quijano using Catwalk by TIGI **Model** Zoey Kay **Makeup Assistant** Alexa Taylor **Photography Assistant** Indigo Rohrer **Nails** Zaida Ibrahim-Gani using Essie

Next page **Makeup** Kryolan Supracolor 079, Icicle Gel, Thickening Agent; MAC Lipstick (Lady Danger) **Photography** Camille Sanson **Hair** Jose Quijano using Catwalk by TIGI **Model** Karina White **Makeup Assistant** Alexa Taylor **Photography Assistant** Indigo Rohrer

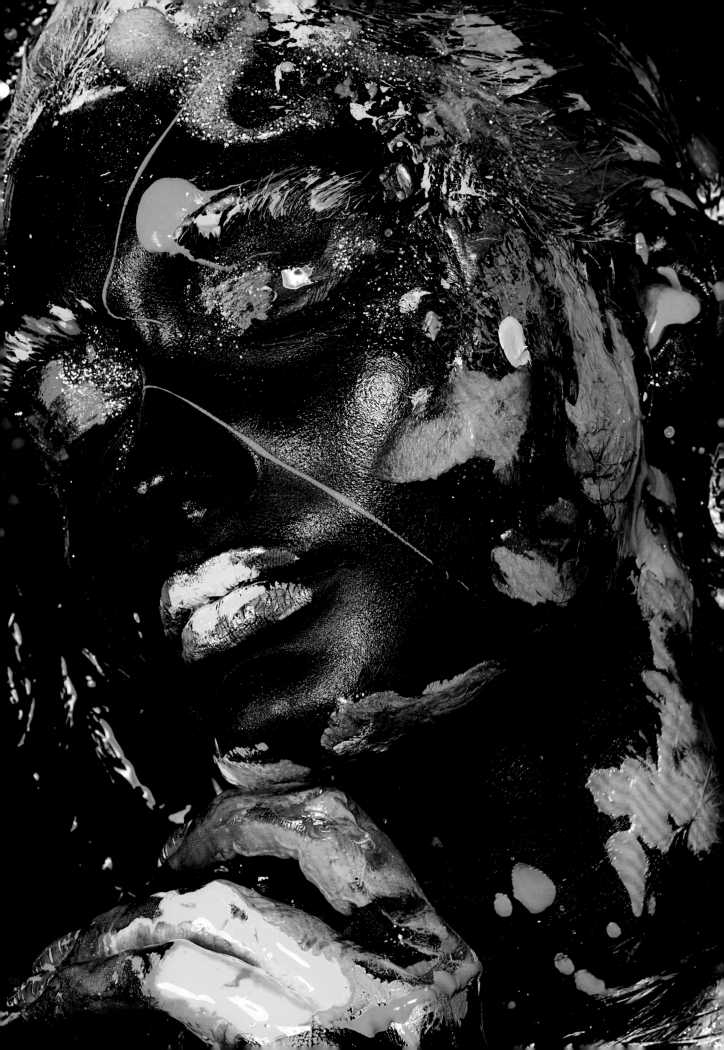

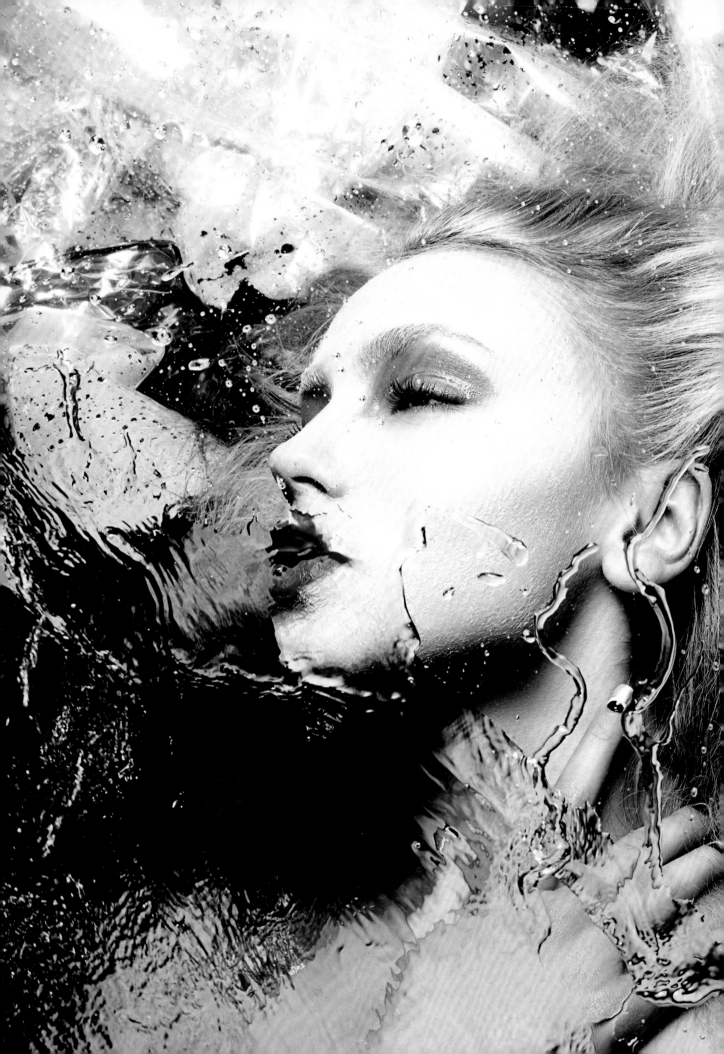

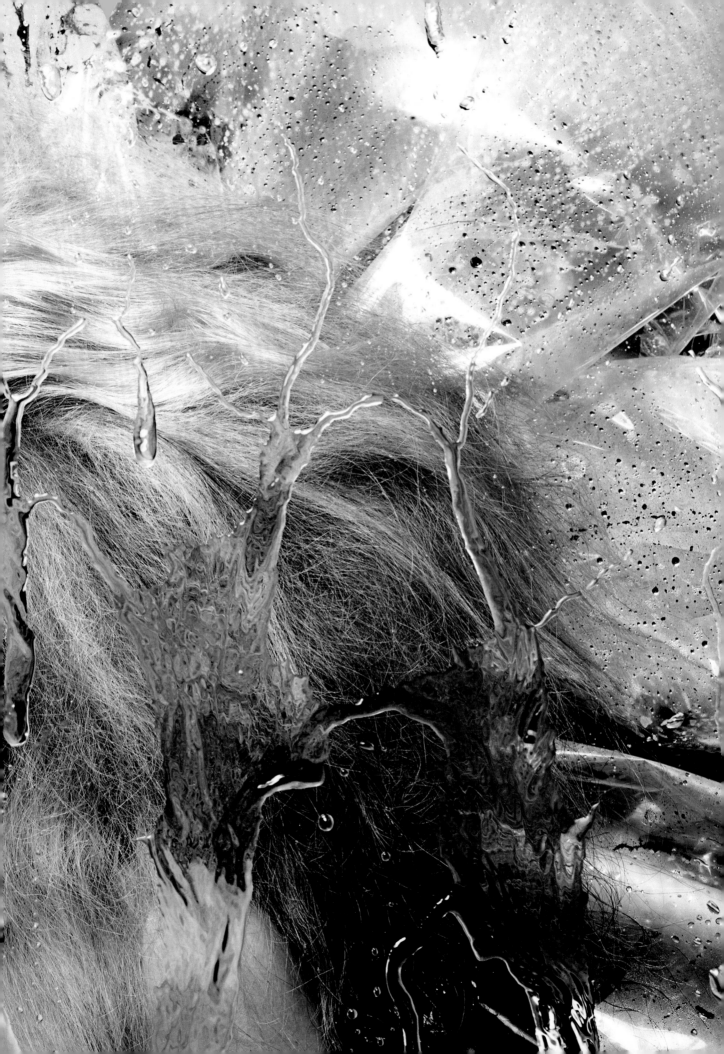

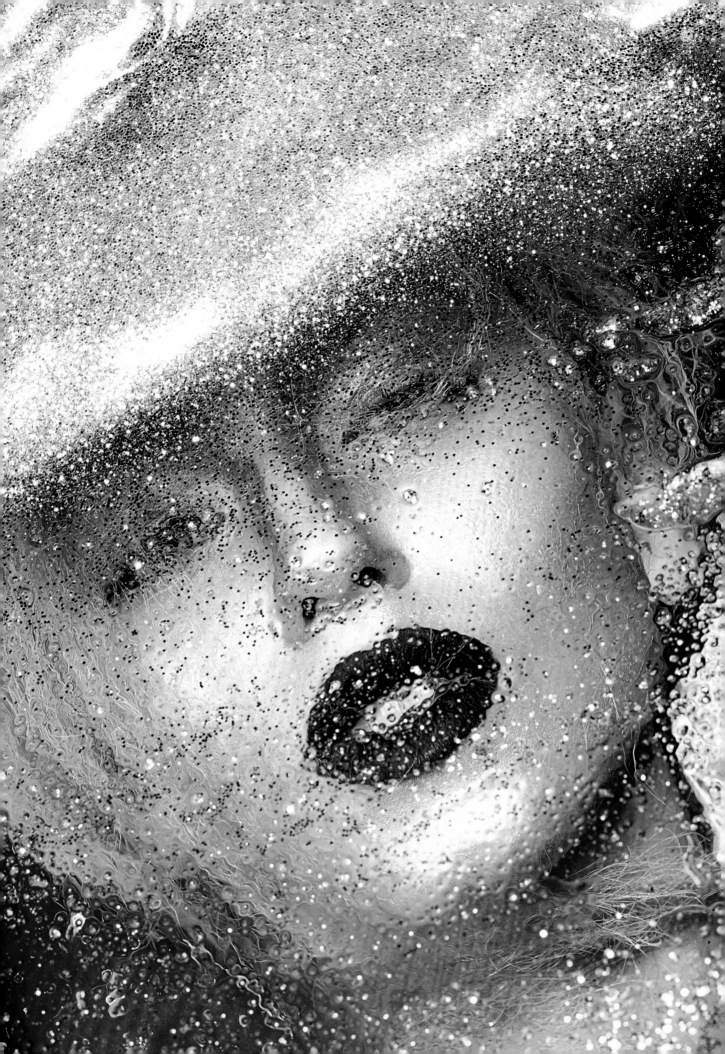

Left **Makeup** Kryolan Supracolor Palette 24 Colors K (Silver, Black), HD Micro Foundation Palette, Make-Up Blend, Liquid Glitter, Dermacolor Fixing Powder **Photography** Camille Sanson **Hair** Jose Quijano using Catwalk by TIGI **Model** Karina White @ Select **Makeup Assistant** Alexa Taylor **Nails** Zaida Ibrahim-Gani using Essie

Below **Makeup** MAC Fluidline (Blacktrack), Pigment (Teal), Studio Face and Body Foundation **Photography** Camille Sanson **Hair and Makeup** team as above **Model** Zoey Kay @ Storm

Next page **Makeup** Kryolan Aquacolor Liquid UV Color Orange, Cream Color Circle UV, Liquid Glitter, Shimmering Event Foundation, Supracolor Shimmering Vision Palette; MAC Pigments (Rock It Yellow, Clear Sky Blue); Eldora eyelashes **Photography** Camille Sanson **Hair and Makeup** team as above **Model** Zoey Kay @ Storm

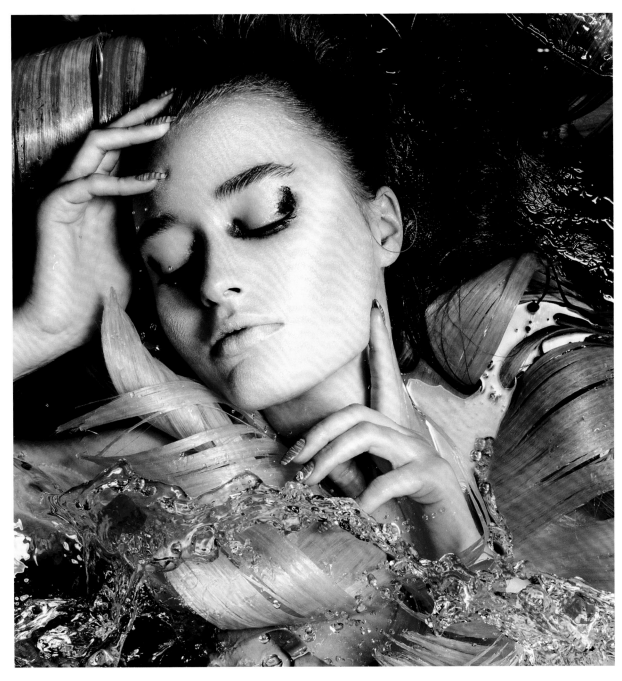

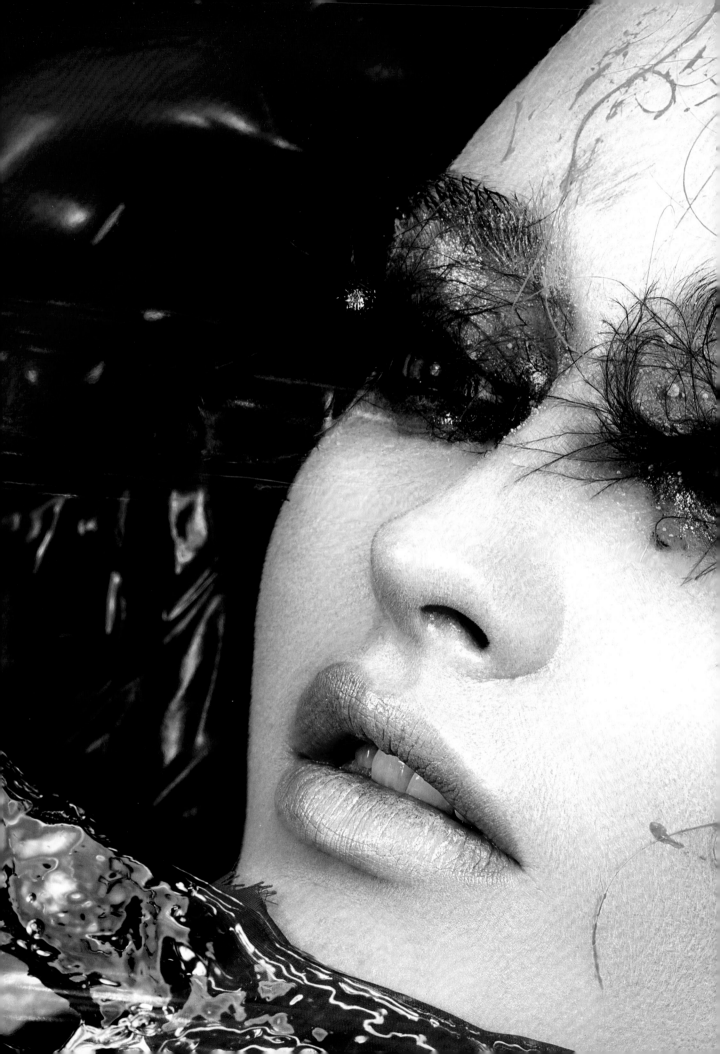

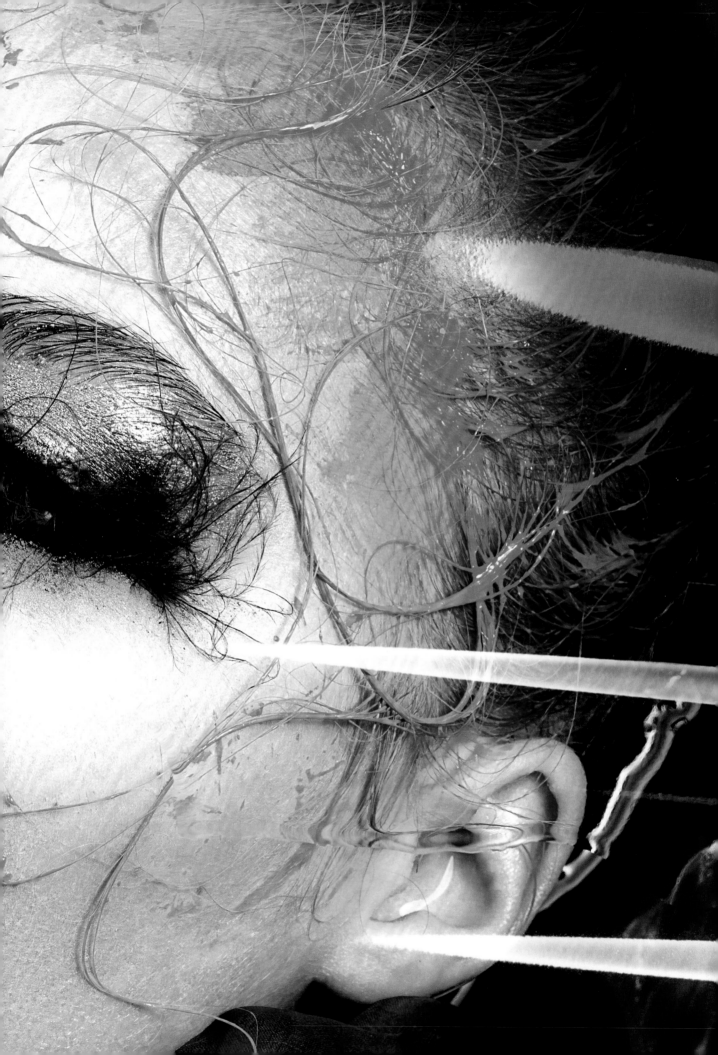

'All art is an abstraction to some degree.'

– Henry Moore (1898-1986)

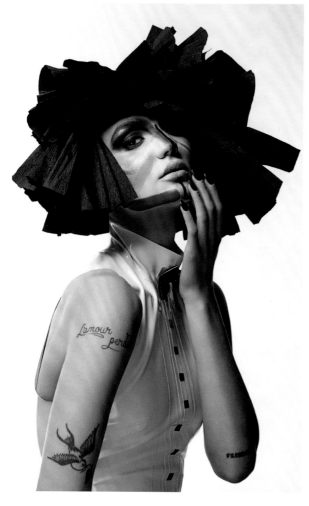

Henry Moore

Yorkshireman Henry Moore's monumental bronze figures undulate like the Dales of his childhood. His abstraction of the human figure is what I have taken inspiration from for these images. I've created organic shapes and voluminous forms on the body, especially in the head area, using metallic styling and with restrictive makeup.

The boldness of the form balances well with the distortion of the facial features through paint and texture. As with Moore, the finished article is a creative expression of a mood. The sculptor favoured the practice of direct carving, letting his toolmarks become part of the finished piece. In the words of Moore himself, 'One mustn't let technique be the consciously important thing. It should be at the service of expressing the form.'

Above **Makeup** (see p.202) **Photography** Camille Sanson **Hair** Diana Moar **Nails** Pebbles Aikens using Essie

Opposite **Makeup** MAC Studio Face and Body Foundation (White), Full Coverage Foundation (White), Sheertone Blush (Pinch O' Peach), Eye Shadow (White Frost), Eye Pencil (Fascinating); Swarovski Crystals **Photography** Camille Sanson **Hair** Diana Moar **Jacket** Ashley Isham **Model** Ellie

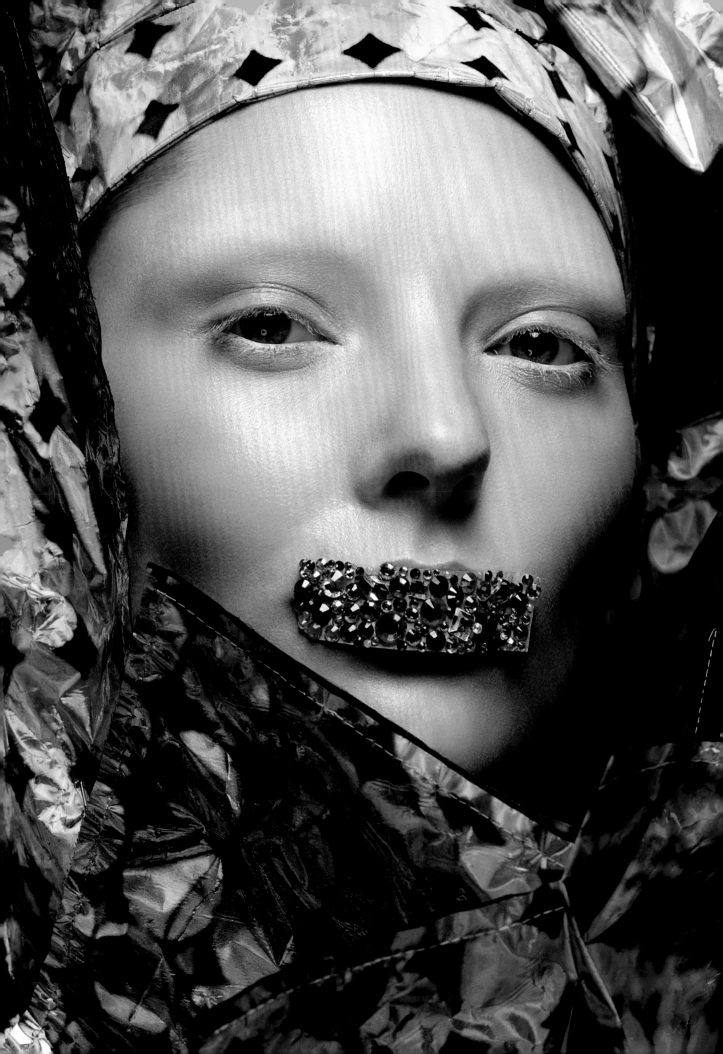

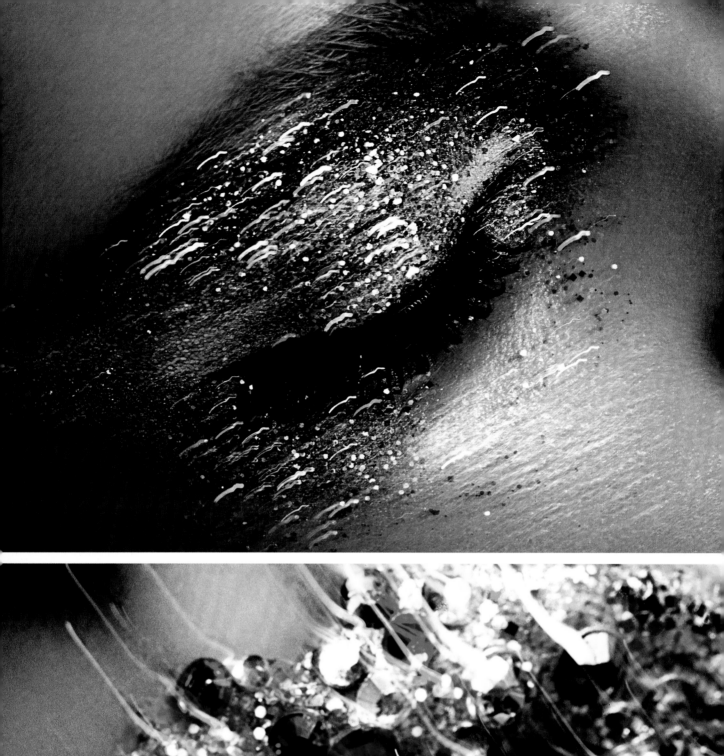
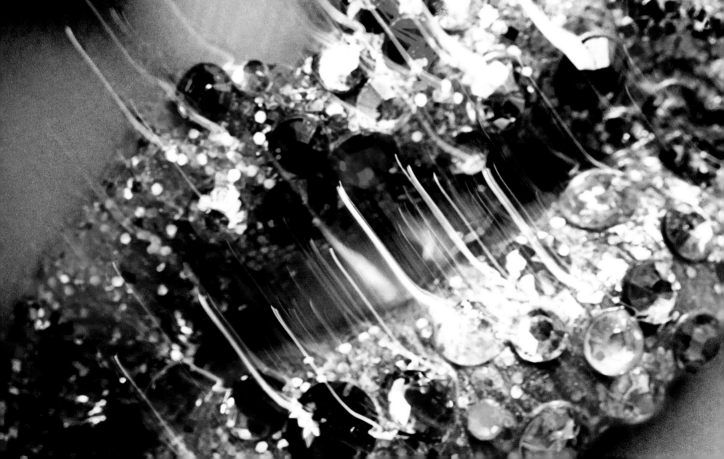

'*The difference between art about death and actual death is that one's a celebration and the other's a dull fact*'.

– Damien Hirst (b. 1965)

Damien Hirst

From the age of 16, when he would make a pilgrimage to the anatomy department of Leeds School of Medicine in order to draw corpses, Damien Hirst has been preoccupied with the major themes of life, death and art. He's the man behind some of the most sensational pieces in contemporary art – notably his shark piece *The Physical Impossibility of Death in the Mind of Someone Living* (1991), which was unveiled as part of the Saatchi Gallery's 1992 *Young British Artists* exhibition. As the artist joked, 'It's amazing what you can do with an E in A-level art, a twisted imagination and a chainsaw.'

It was major themes of life and death – particularly *For The Love Of God* from 2007, a platinum skull encrusted with 8,601 flawless diamonds and human teeth – that inspired the image on the next pages. Its message of 'victory over decay' is a beautiful one, and it's unusual that the raw materials of art are so precious in themselves. I wanted to portray that feeling in an image.

To create the final image I played down the model's features with matt black paint, creating a hollow emptiness to imply skull-like features. Using a bespoke crystal headpiece designed in the shape of a skull by hair stylist Marc Eastlake, I then added more texture with paint glitter and individual Swarovski crystals to complement the shape and outline of the face. Capturing the movement of the head in slow motion on camera allowed me to distort the image and elongate the head, which also brought out the colour and shine.

Top **Makeup** MAC Glitter (Smolder), Strobe Cream, Studio Face and Body Foundation, Penultimate Eye Liner (Rapidblack), Haute & Naughty Lash, 6 Lash eyelashes **Photography** Mark Cant **Model** Ellie

Left **Makeup** MAC Pro Longwear Lip Pencil (More to Love), Cremesheen Lipstick (Lickable), Glitter (Reflects Pearl, 3D Silver); Swarovski Crystals

Following page **Makeup** MAC Greasepaint Stick, Glitter (3D Silver, Red), Mixing Medium **Photography** Catherine Harbour **Headpiece** Mark Eastlake using Swarovski **Model** Rae Matthews @ Nevs

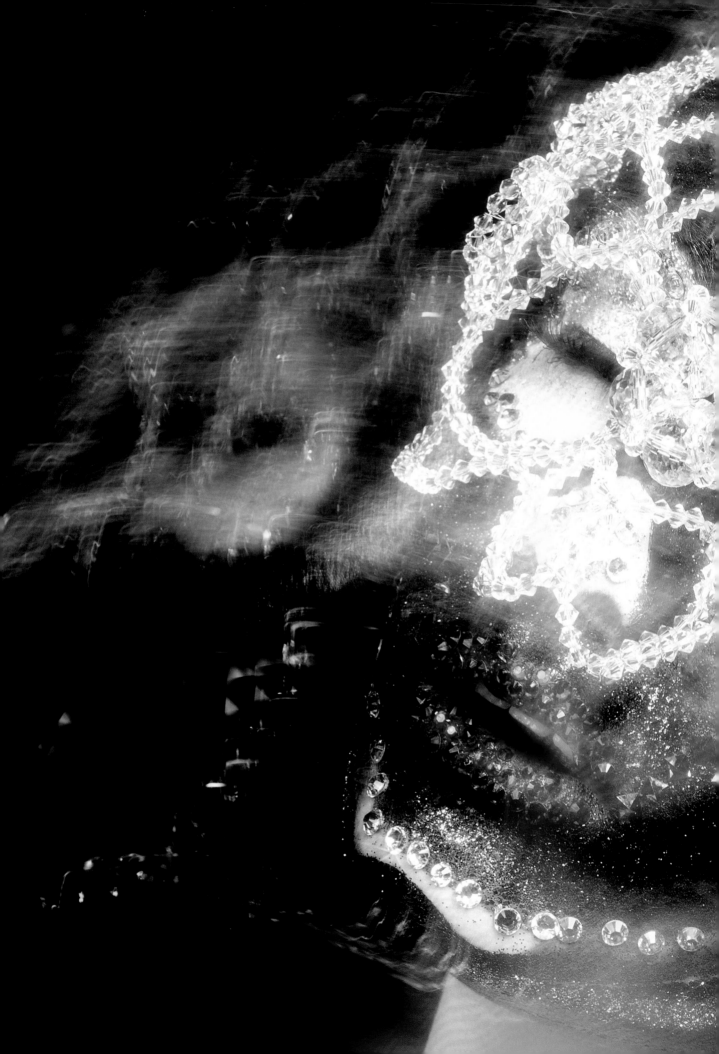

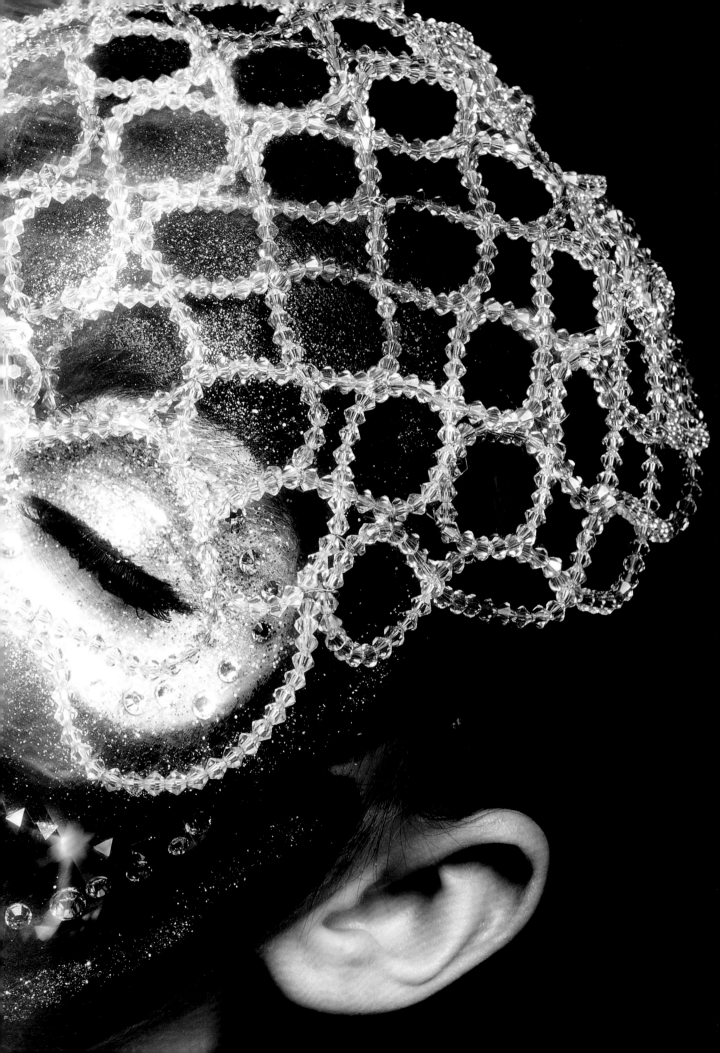

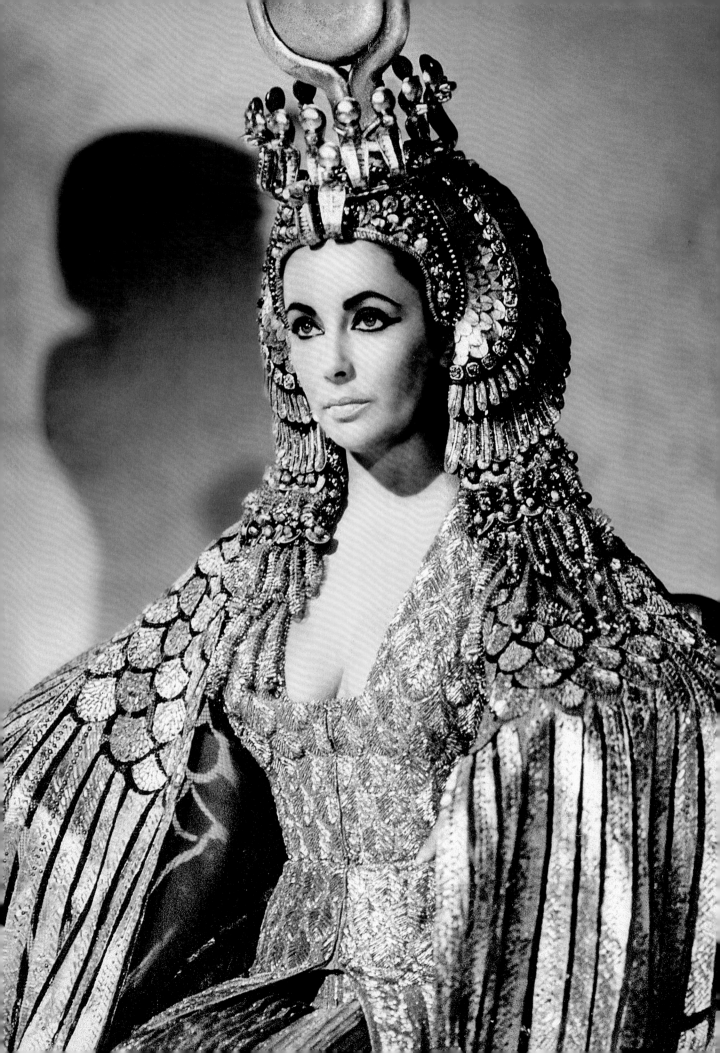

3. Cinema & TV

Cleopatra, The Tudors, Marie Antoinette, Downton Abbey, Gosford Park, The Great Gatsby, Mad Men, Charlie's Angels, Dallas, Edward Scissorhands, Sin City

---

'Creating fantasy and bringing dreams to life is possible with a little teamwork.'

'As with a magician, not all tricks
are revealed, but with the stroke of
a brush and a creative imagination,
who knows what magic can happen.'

Cleopatra

When putting together a moodboard for a photoshoot, the worlds of film and television provide a wealth of inspiration for the fashion industry's makeup artists. In this chapter I look at some of the screen's most trendsetting costume looks from popular shows and films of the last few decades. Using these as a reference point I showcase my interpretations of these beauty styles with one iconic and cinematic image for each era.

As far back as I can remember, I loved watching Elizabeth Taylor playing the beautiful pharaoh Cleopatra in this 1963 epic by Joseph L. Mankiewicz. I wanted to bring her signature heavily kohl-lined eyes and brows to my image, but also add in a golden richness through accessories and a headdress to give the model that 'goddess' feel. So, using my own style I created gold, glitter-textured skin – even down to her hands, which were outlined like a golden glove. The pointing hand represents the regal nature of the subject. In the film the look is more glamorous and bold, whereas I have taken a more avant-garde approach. If Cleopatra bathed in milk to look beautiful, I'm certain she would have loved to have been seen encrusted in gold glitter! The ancient Egyptians believed that cosmetics had magical powers, and to this day Cleopatra's various graphic, winged eyeliner shapes are often referenced across the industry, from catwalk shows to editorial features. The original 'mineral' makeup, vibrant green eyeshadow was made from the copper compound malachite, while dazzling cobalt blue was made from lapis lazuli.

Makeup Kyrolan Supracolor Shimmering Vision Palette, Aquacolor B and FP, Polyester Glimmer (Gold) in fine, medium and large **Photography** Camille Sanson **Hair** Diana Moar **Styling** Karl Willett **Jewellery** Erickson Beamon **Model** Claudia Devlin @ Premier **Makeup Assistant** Lolo Page **Photography Assistant** Indigo Rohrer **Nails** Pebbles Aikens using Minx

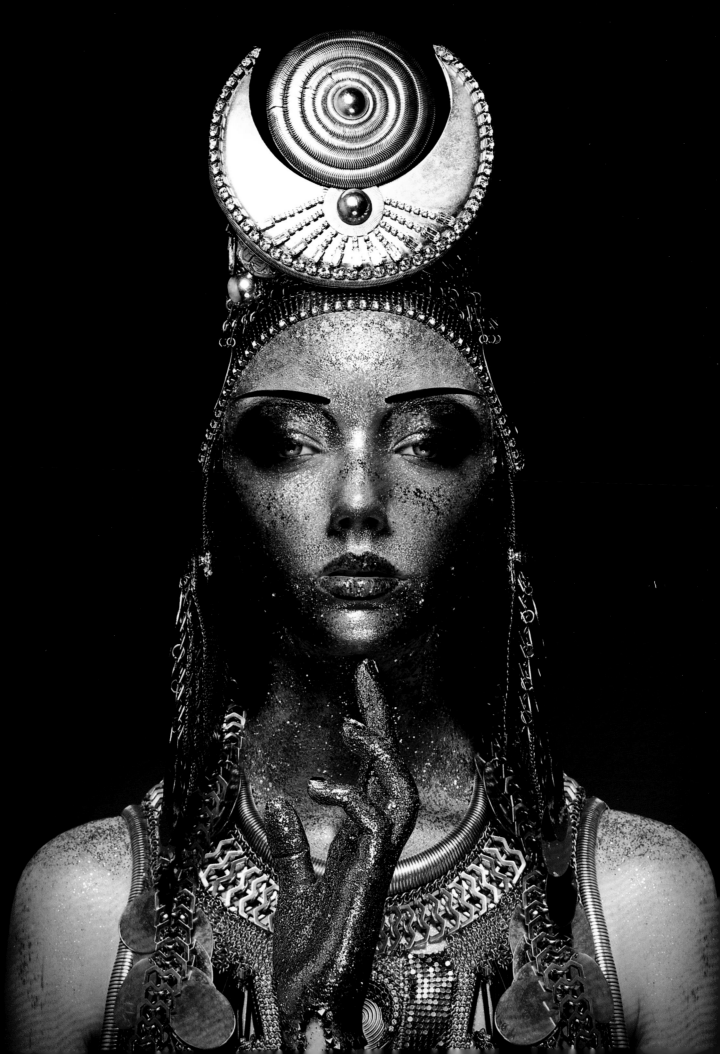

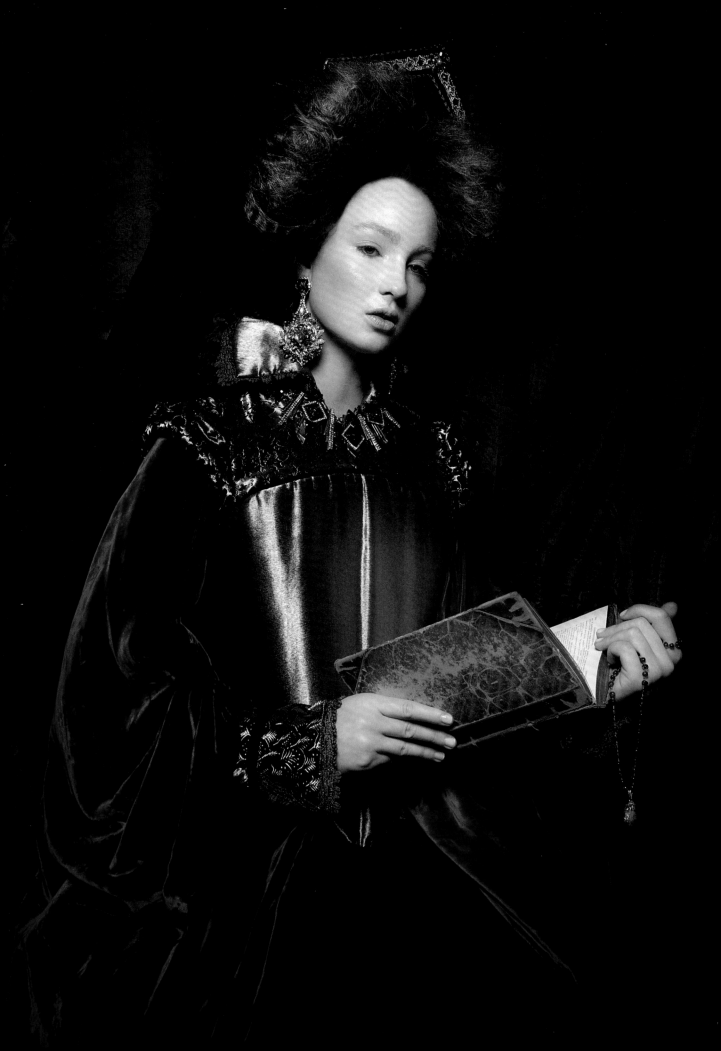

'Like costume designers, makeup artists are storytellers. The relationship between hair stylists and makeup artists is a huge part of what brings any shoot to life. Makeup and hair really helps the audience to understand that what they see on the page is real.'

– Diana Moar, Hair Stylist

The Tudors

Opposite **Makeup** Kryolan Shimmering Event Foundation (Pearl), Make Up Blend, HD Micro Foundation TV White; MAC Lipstick (Show Orchid Amplified Creme); Daniel Sandler Watercolour Fluid Blusher (Cherub) **Photography** Camille Sanson **Hair** Diana Moar **Styling** Karl Willett **Jewellery** Erickson Beamon **Costume** National Theatre Costume **Model** Rose Ellis @ Storm **Hair Assistant** Karl Willett **Makeup Assistant** Loan Nguyen **Photography Assistant** Laurie Noble **Styling Assistants** Adele Pentland and Harry Clements

Next page **Makeup** Kryolan Shimmering Event Foundation (Pearl), TV Paint Stick (TV White), Make Up Blend, Lip and Cheek (Lotus), Eye Shadow Iridescent (Golden Pink); The Body Shop Shimmer Cube Palette (26, Hot Pink), Divide & Multiply Mascara; Benefit Speed Brow, POREfessional, That Gal Brightening Face Primer **Photography** Camille Sanson **Set Design** Louis Mariette **Flowers** Wildabout Flowers (www.wildaboutflowers.co.uk) **Millinery**/bejewelled headpieces/sculpture heads (Louis Mariette) **Costumes** (from left to right) 1. dress (Sorapol); 2. blue lace dress (Dolce & Gabbana), boots (Vivian Ying); 3. red lace blouse (Sorapol); 4. blue dress (Sorapol), shoes (Gina); 5. black jacket (Sorapol); 6. white dress (National Theatre Costume); 7. blue lace blouse and skirt (Sorapol) **Models** Marta, Rose Ellis, Georgia @ Storm **Styling Assistants** Charles Boyles and Carlos Contreras

The first decade of the new millennium revisited Britain's colourful history from 1485–1603 for the small screen in Michael Hirst's Golden Globe-winning TV show. In the 2007 series, particular attention was paid to the costumes – rich, jewel-like colours in heavy, layered fabrics such as velvet and damask silk, with flamboyant touches such as cloaks and headdresses. My inspiration for this image was the traditional style of portraiture at the time, by artists such as Nicholas Hilliard (1547–1619) and George Gower (1540–1596); the latter was the Serjeant Painter to Queen Elizabeth I and painted her as an ethereal, commanding beauty set against dark-hued, grandiose backgrounds. To create my image I chose to work with the traditional makeup look of alabaster powdered skin. I started by blanking out the features, then used cheek stains for a natural, rosy glow, which I built up in sheer layers to keep it transparent. A faint, stained lip adds to the natural look – it's the simplicity of the makeup that gives a virginal and holy look. There's a real two-dimensional drama to the Tudor paintings, which we recreated with soft candlelight. The girl sits with her tome, lips soft, her face expressionless – a moment in which she is lost in pious contemplation.

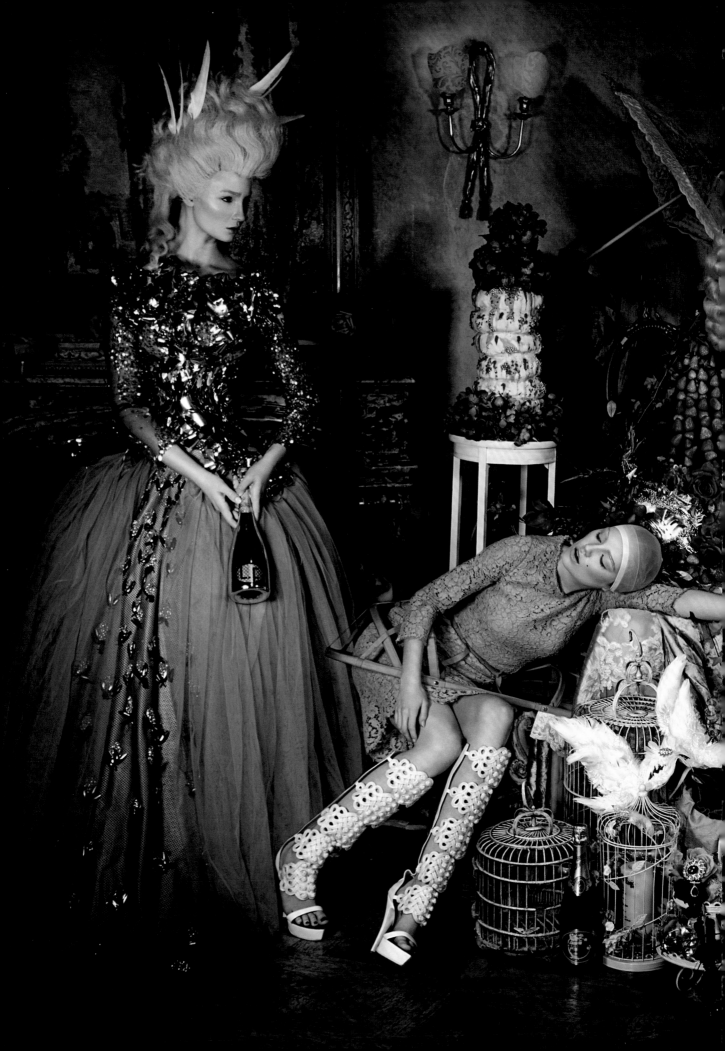

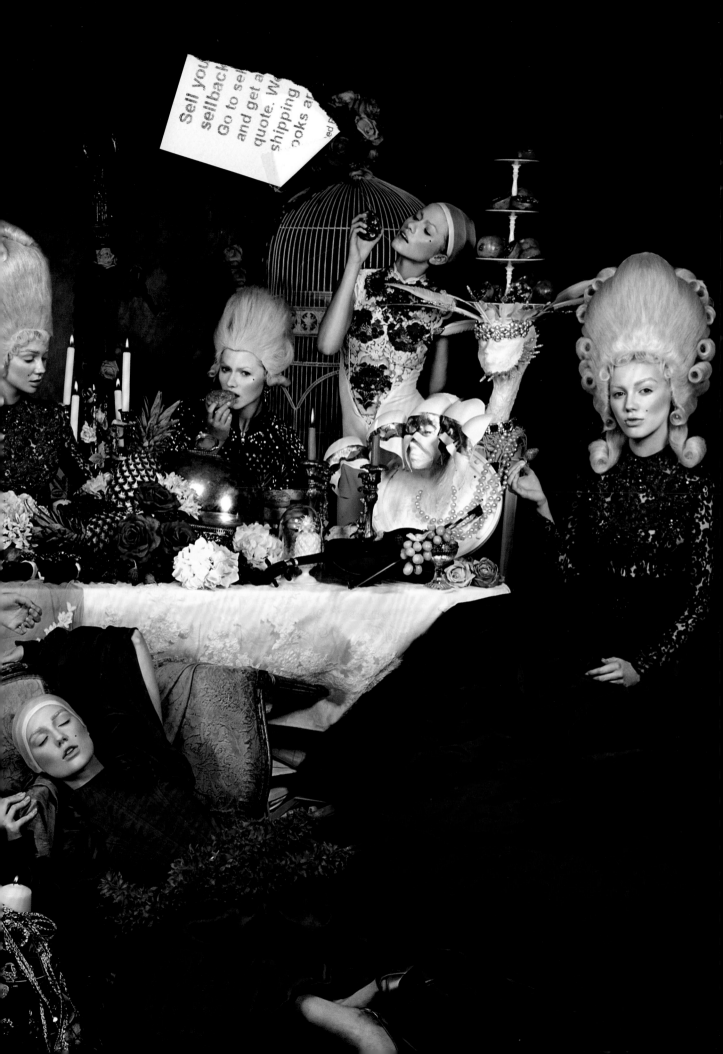

Marie Antoinette

Downton Abbey

Director Sofia Coppola's 2006 take on French Rococo opulence saw Kirsten Dunst own the role of the ill-fated queen. Inspiration for the image on the previous pages was taken from the young queen's lavishly hedonistic dinner parties that were full of colour and laden with fancy cakes and inviting platters of fruit – a veritable banquet of lovely things. I really went to town with the bouffant hair rolls, extra-pale skin, rouged cheeks, beauty spots and flamboyant styling. The paler the skin on the model, the more like a porcelain doll she would look. I next added washes of strong pastels, and a real emphasis on the big hair. The pale, powdered skin is ultra-feminine and layered with deep purple and pink tones of blush powder to create an air of childlike innocence. The lip colour is more of a stain, with no defined edges but depth in the very centre, as if she had just bitten a cherry. This doll-like look appears season after season on the catwalks and is popular for couture shows and magazine editorials.

The restrained beauty of the Edwardian era was recreated to global acclaim in Julian Fellowes' lavish TV series. *Downton Abbey*, in general, was quite simple and neutral with its makeup, so I took inspiration from Michelle Dockery's character Lady Mary Crawley. She was always elegant and groomed from morning to night – changing outfits for every social occasion. My model was dark haired and stunning without makeup, so I played with more elaborate hair and shifted the focus to her reflection in the mirror, where you can see her radiant, pale skin, youthfully smooth and defined, with an English rose flush on the cheeks and softly rounded lips. I wanted to create something haunting and beautifully simple. In the background the maid is still groomed but plainer, her matt skin has only a dash of translucent powder. She stares poignantly into the distance as 'Lady Mary' dresses in opulent silk for dinner, holding herself with an air of authority. The image is kept rigid and formal to reflect the class structure of those times. The image takes on an editorial quality, with saturated tones and carefully considered composition.

Makeup Lancôme Miracle Air de Teint, Hypnôse Mascara, Contour Pro, L'Absolu Nu Lipstick (205, Beige Charnel); HD Brows
Photography Camille Sanson **Clothes** (left) black dress (Dolce & Gabbana), apron (National Theatre costume); (right) gown (Reem Juan)
Models Marta, Rose Ellis @ Storm

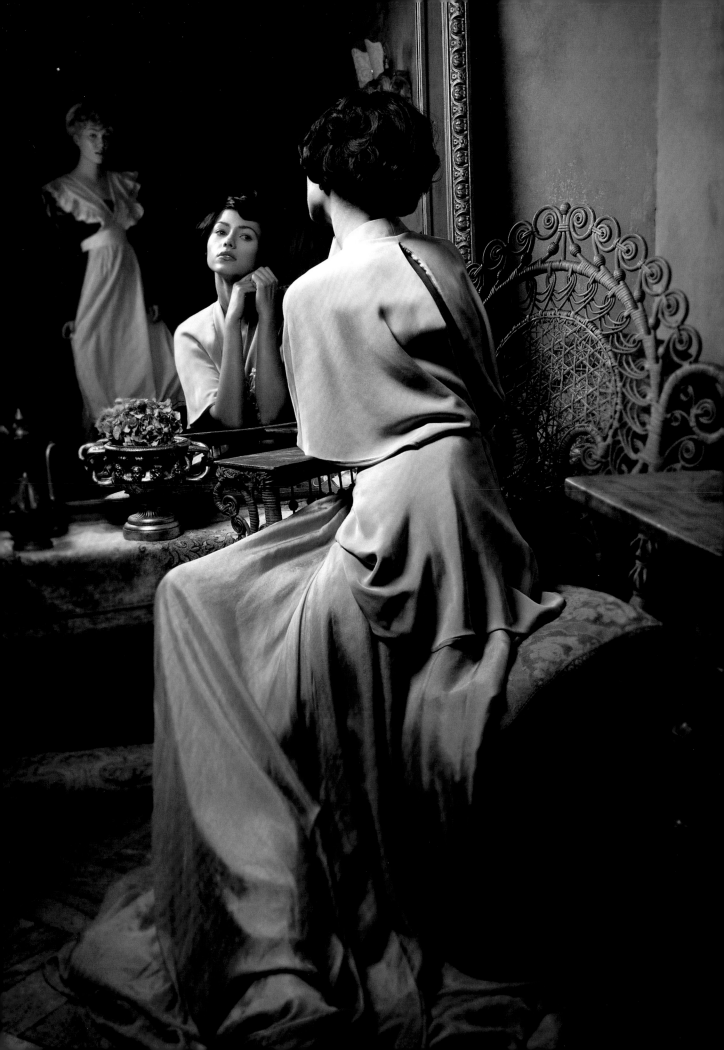

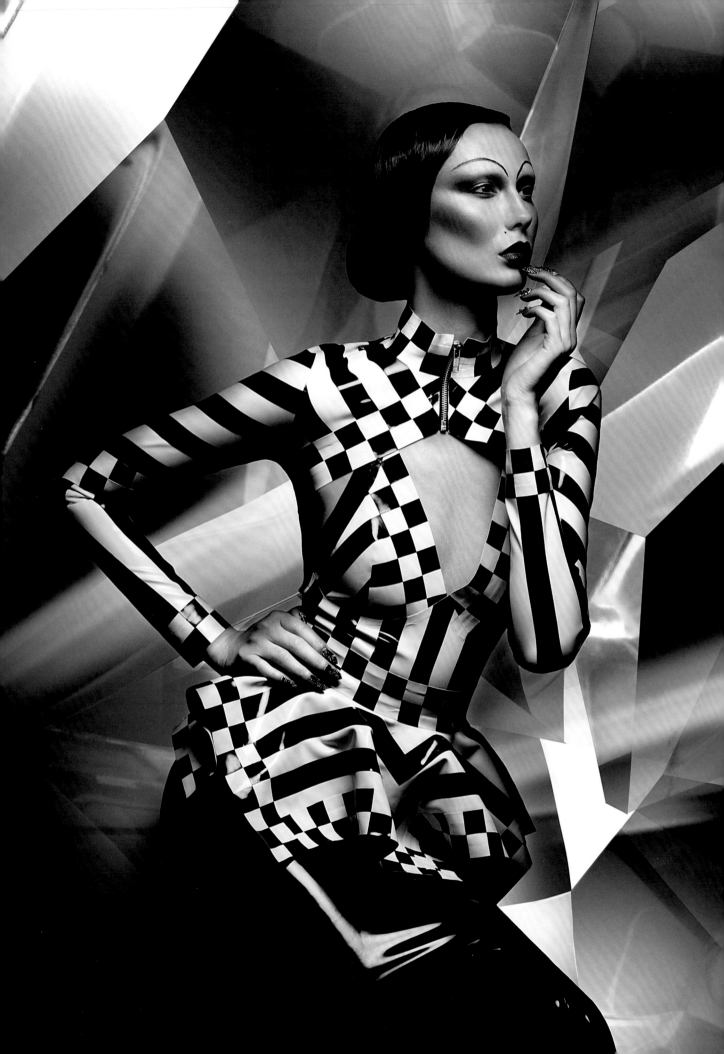

'Fashion fades, style dies, art remains.'
– Daniel Lismore, Fashion Stylist

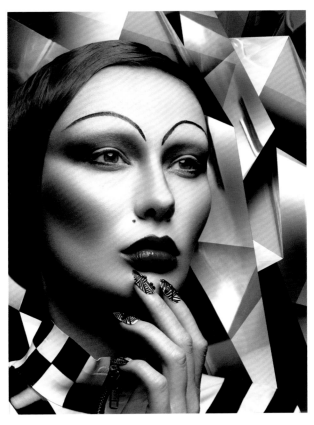

Gosford Park

A murder mystery and the 1930s British class system are the themes of this 2001 movie. The industrial 1930s saw the bold, geometric shapes of the Art Deco era flourish – both in architecture and painting, such as the graphic facial contours of women depicted by leading artists such as Thomas Benton. *Gosford Park* toyed with the theme of class division, specifically the notion of upstairs/downstairs in a household – the privileged lives of aristocrats set against those of their army of servants. It was an age of glamour – hair was immaculate and perfectly coiffed close to the head, and the makeup was flawless. All the features were defined – perfectly arched, thin eyebrows and sharply defined, bright red lips set against heavily pigmented eyes, sockets darkened to create shape. Highlighter and contouring were added to exaggerate the cheekbones. Today the look epitomizes the vintage glamour style made popular by burlesque dancers such as Dita Von Teese.

Makeup Kryolan Cine-Wax, TV Paint Stick, Eye Shadow Palettes (Variety, Metallique)
Photography Camille Sanson **Hair** Diana Moar using Bumble and Bumble **Styling** Karl Willett **Clothes** William Wilde **Model** Lakiza
Photography Assistant Indigo Rohrer **Nails** The Freelance Workspace using VuDu Nails

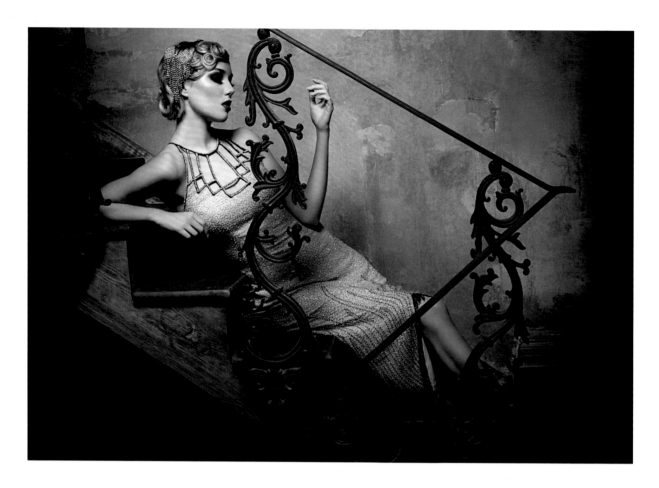

The Great Gatsby

The twenties roared even louder at the hands of
Baz Luhrmann in the 2013 movie based on F. Scott
Fitzgerald's classic novel. The aftermath of World
War II was a dynamic and modern time, which saw
women win the vote, dance halls filled with jazz
music, and the beginning of the cult of celebrity.
I wanted to reference the decadent glamour and
create an intimate image with strong emphasis on
hair, makeup and diamond accessories. In contrast
with the Edwardian era's subtle makeup and long
hair, I exaggerated the makeup with dramatic shades
of oyster and silver, adding the coral pink and lilac
that were key in the Art Deco palette. My focus was
on a smoky, sultry, round eye, paired with rich
burgundy-toned matt lips to keep it contemporary.
In the film itself the statement was made with
the classic short hair of the period and bejewelled
headbands rather than a strong lip colour. This era is
often a reference point for beauty on the catwalk, and
for many editorial shoots. The glamour and
dramatically contrasting makeup makes a strong
statement that oozes sex appeal and rebellion.

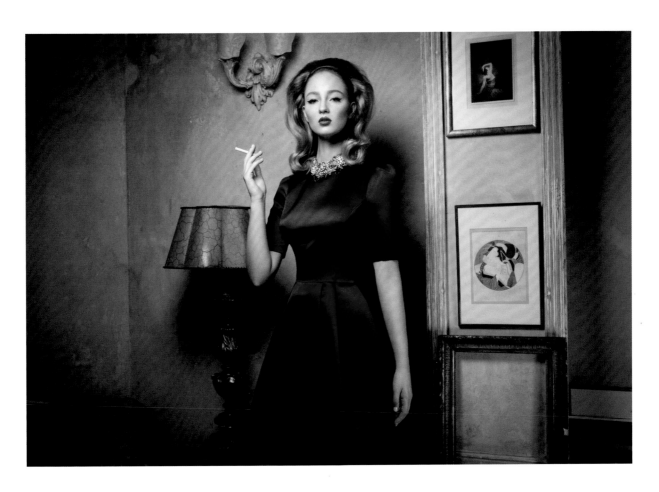

Mad Men

Opposite **Makeup** Bourjois Eyes Smoky Stories (Ocean Obsession), Rouge Edition Velvet Lipstick (01, Personne ne rouge), Mega Liner (Black), Délice de Poudre Duo, Blush (34, Rose d'Or), Volume 1-Seconde Mascara (Ultra Black), Full Volume Mascara **Photography** Camille Sanson **Hair** Diana Moar **Styling** Karl Willett **Headpiece** Louis Mariette **Dress** National Theatre Costume **Model** Georgia @ Storm **Makeup Assistant** Loan Nguyen **Photography Assistant** Laurie Noble **Styling Assistants** Adele Pentland and Harry Clements

Above **Makeup** NARS Radiant Cream Compact Foundation, Velvet Matte Lip Pencil (Dragon Girl); Daniel Sandler Sculpt and Slim; Yves Saint Laurent Shocking False Lash Effect Eyeliner; Eyelure 101 Lashes; HD Brows **Photography** Camille Sanson **Hair** Diana Moar **Styling** Karl Willett **Dress** Suzannah **Model** Joy @ Storm **Makeup Assistant** Lolo Page **Styling Assistants** Adele Pentland and Harry Clements

Matthew Weiner's contemporary TV series, set in the heady world of 1960s advertising, brought 'sexy' back. The sixties saw women beginning to climb to positions of power – but they did it with cinched waists, conical brassières and kitten heels. In this shot I emphasized the eyes with black, feline flicks of eyeliner, bold red lips and silky bouffant hair. The other side of makeup in the '60s was the wide-eyed, false-lashed British Mod look, as personified by Twiggy. The version that I have created here is more akin to the classic Hitchcock look, but with added editorial gloss and a statement hairband. The black eyeliner/red lip combination is perennially fashionable, and it's a look that works well for the glamour of the red carpet. Here it's also paired with a contoured eye in taupe shadow, lashings of mascara and a defined brow.

Charlie's Angels

The classic 1970s detective show remains a key reference point for that decade's glamorous beauty looks. Like Farrah Fawcett's signature flicks, this look is all about the wonderful, luscious hair and blended, smoky eyeshadow. The look is typified by bronzed, sun-kissed skin and makeup that is simple but has warm, golden tones mixed with mid-grey to brown tones.

Clashing a gorgeous, sexy red lip with a satin finish adds glamour. Golden tones are used to highlight the cheekbones for a very strong contoured cheek, but when the light hits her face you can see an angelic softness. The idea was to create a strong, iconic image that oozed effortless femininity and a strong beauty – on catwalks, and swimwear shoots in particular, the '70s look is often used to give an edgy, powerful attitude, although if the model already has the tanned body and face often only a statement eyebrow or lip is needed with a little contouring. For a more high-octane, disco look, use a bleached brow and metallic eyeshadow.

Makeup Giorgio Armani Luminous Silk Foundation, Eyes to Kill Eyeshadow Quad, Eye & Brow Maestro, Smooth Silk Eye Pencil, Eyes to Kill Mascara, Lip Maestro 503 Red Fuchsia **Photography** Catherine Harbour **Hair** Chie Sato using Label.m **Model** Zoe @ MOT Models **Makeup Assistant** Eoin Whelan

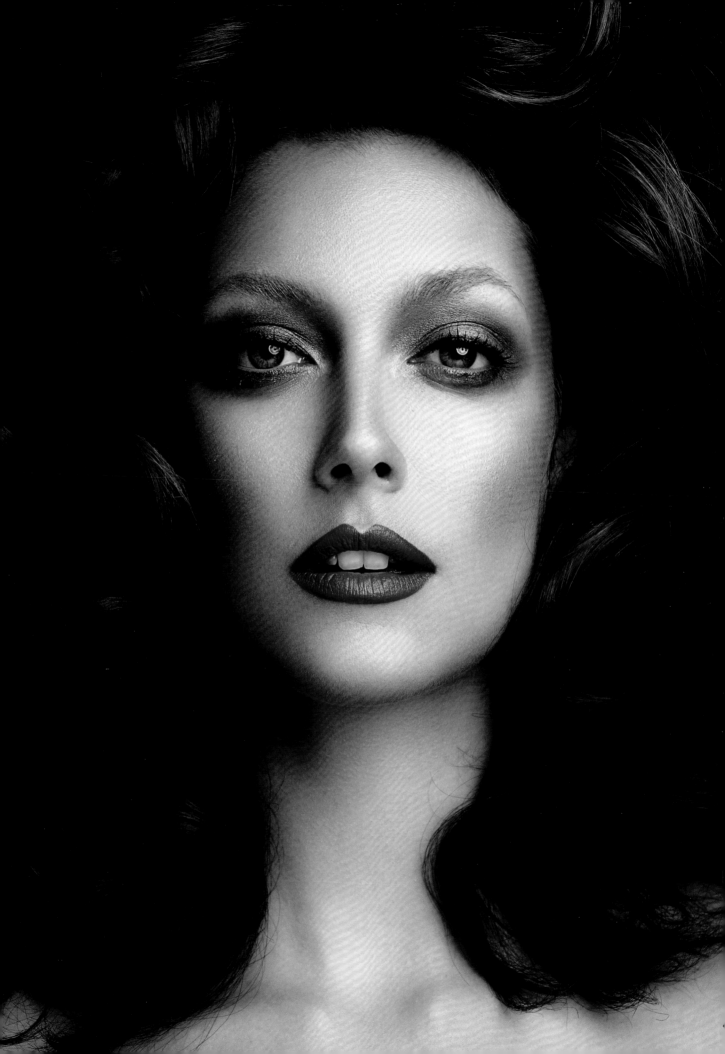

'Hair can never be too big nor heels too high.'

– William Wilde, Designer and Costumier

Dallas

This period was all about maximalism. Big shoulders, bold accessories, bright colours – blues, yellows and greens, gold eyes with contrasting lipstick of deep, blood-red mixed with pink. Topped off with glitter! Even the hair is ostentatious with a big, wafting side-fringe. The look is then styled with oversized chandelier earrings and yet more colour from the boxy, fuchsia power suit. The key is to balance all the competitive elements so that it looks fabulous rather than kitsch; just think of Joan Collins in her voluminous, off-the-shoulder dresses in chocolate-wrapper metallics. Makeup is top-heavy on the eyes, with thick lashes and mascara. I have incorporated some of the more directional techniques from the '80s into my everyday makeup now, such as using a diluted wash of purple swept up on the cheekbones to the hairline, to provide highlighting and give a fresh and modern twist to the skin.

Makeup Yves Saint Laurent Top Secrets All-in-One BB Cream, Le Teint Touche Éclat Foundation, Blush Radiance, Poudre Compacte Radiance, Couture Palette (Lumieres Majorelle), Rouge Pur Couture 1 Le Rouge, Rouge Laque Vernis à Lèvres Glossy Stain (Rouge Laque), Shocking False Lash Effect Eyeliner, Long-Lasting Eye Pencil, Baby Doll Mascara; Eyelure Naturalites Natural Volume Lashes **Photography** Camille Sanson **Hair** Diana Moar **Styling** Karl Willett **Clothes** jumpsuit (Beyond Retro), belt (Moschino) **Jewellery** Liz Mendez Vintage **Model** Georgia @ Storm **Makeup Assistant** Loan Nguyen **Photography Assistant** Laurie Noble **Styling Assistant** Adele Pentland and Harry Clements

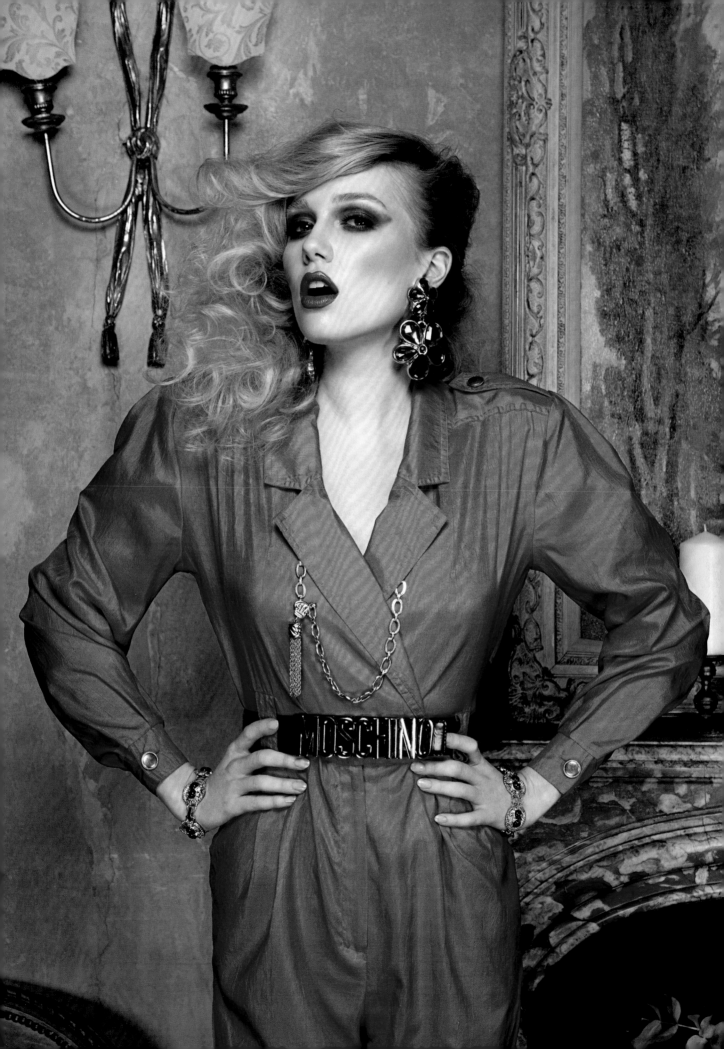

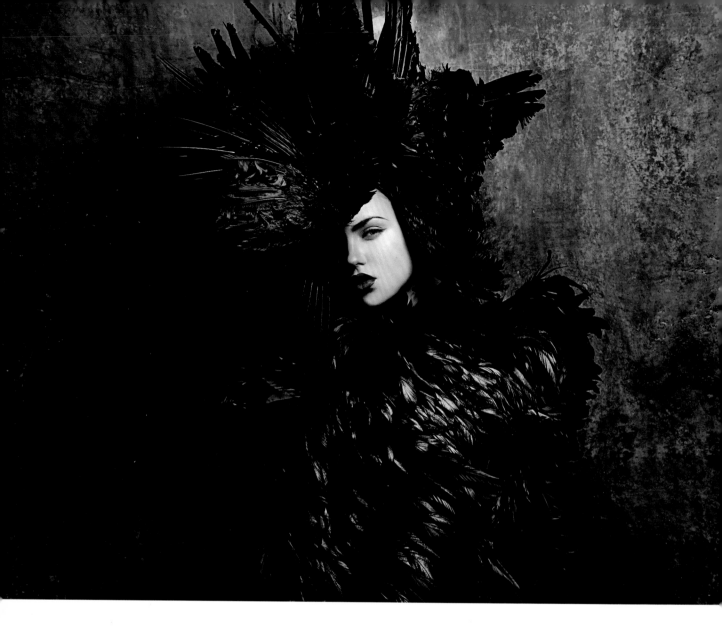

Edward Scissorhands

Dark romantic fantasy is given a dose of 90s
minimalism in Tim Burton's masterpiece from 1990.
The film tells the tale of a gentle but misunderstood
boy who is alienated for being different, and the idea
in the photography was to create a look that told a
story of abandonment, innocence and loneliness. The
'scissor hands' were reinterpreted as unnaturally
long nails. In the film there are the scars and gaunt
contouring on Johnny Depp's Edward character,
which I translated to our female version. Plum tones
and charcoal shades with lashes on top and bottom
gave a wide-eyed sadness, while the skin is kept flat
and matt with a slightly paler skin tone than needed
to bleach out the skin. Contouring using ashy, taupe
colours that were well blended right up to the hairline
give the 'no makeup' effect.

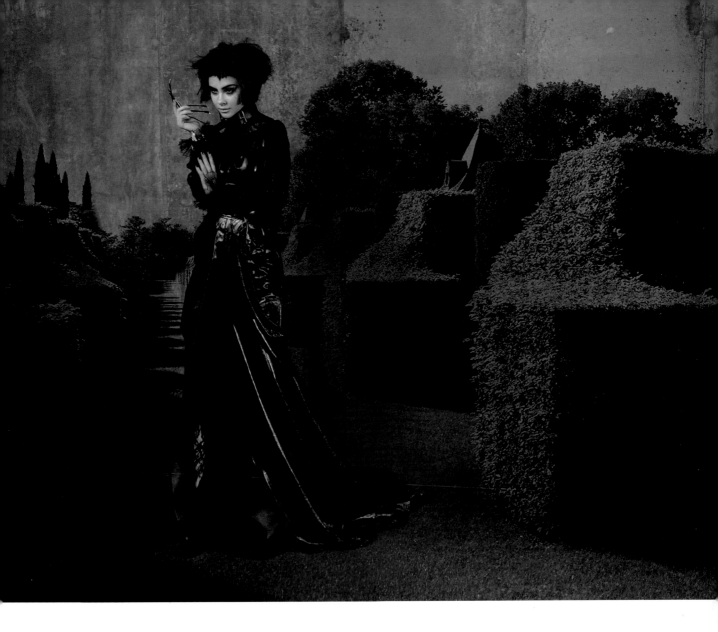

Makeup Kryolan Shimmering Event Foundation (Pearl), HD Micro Foundation TV White; Make Up For Ever 12 Flash Color Case; MAC Pearlglide Intense Eye Liner (Petrol Blue), Fluidline (Blacktrack) **Photography** Camille Sanson **Hair** Diana Moar **Styling** Karl Willett **Makeup Assistant** Kerry White **Styling Assistant** Adele Pentland **Nails** Pebbles Aikens

Left **Hat** Jay Briggs **Cape** Karl Willett **Model** Karina @ Select

Above **Blouse** Dolce & Gabbana **Bra** William Wilde **Skirt** Sorapol **Lace Catsuit** Agent Provocateur **Shoes** Charlene x Sadie **Model** Lidiia @ Leni's

Sin City

Sin City is a highly stylized film noir for the modern age. For the look on the following pages I took my lead from this graphic-novel inspired film, fusing fantasy with reality to create the 'Heroes of Fashion' – a portrayal of the creatives behind the scenes, who collaborate, like a team of unsung superheroes, to create the beautiful images that we see in magazines. The team comprises: the photographer, the hair stylist, the makeup artist, the writer and director. The story behind the image is based on the idea that the 'Heroes' have tried to create a new goddess, the ultimate perfect model, through hair, makeup and styling. The inspiration for their looks is representative of the part they play in the scene. The writer, perched on the chair, is glamorous with a 1960s feel – feline flicks, red lips and immaculately set hair. The hair stylist has a slightly wacky and adventurous hairstyle, with bold eyes and lips. The makeup artist is sexy and dark, with graphic smoky black eyes and dark lips. The stylist is flamboyantly dressed, of course, but is cutting-edge, with a vampy two-toned red and black lip. Finally the supermodel is portrayed as a natural beauty with perfect, full brows, lip line, and luscious lashes and contouring. Using special effects created by melting plastic and then moulding it to the body, the model is distorted into plastic, futuristic perfection.

Makeup Kryolan Aquacolor Liquid UV Color and Supracolor Palette 24 Colors N and K **Photography** Camille Sanson **Hair** Diana Moar **Styling** Karl Willett **Bodypiece** Justin Smith **Model** Karina @ Select **Makeup Assistant** Kerry White **Styling Assistant** Adele Pentland **Photography Assistant/Set Design** Rua Acorn, Lianna Fouler and Brendan Grealis **Nails** Pebbles Aikens

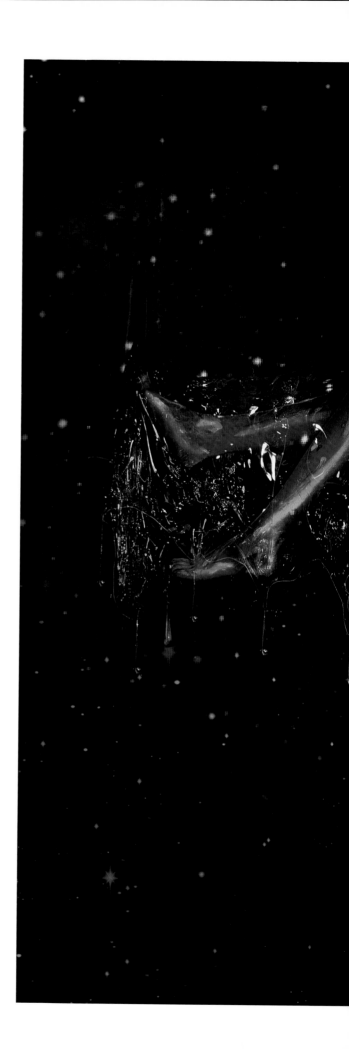

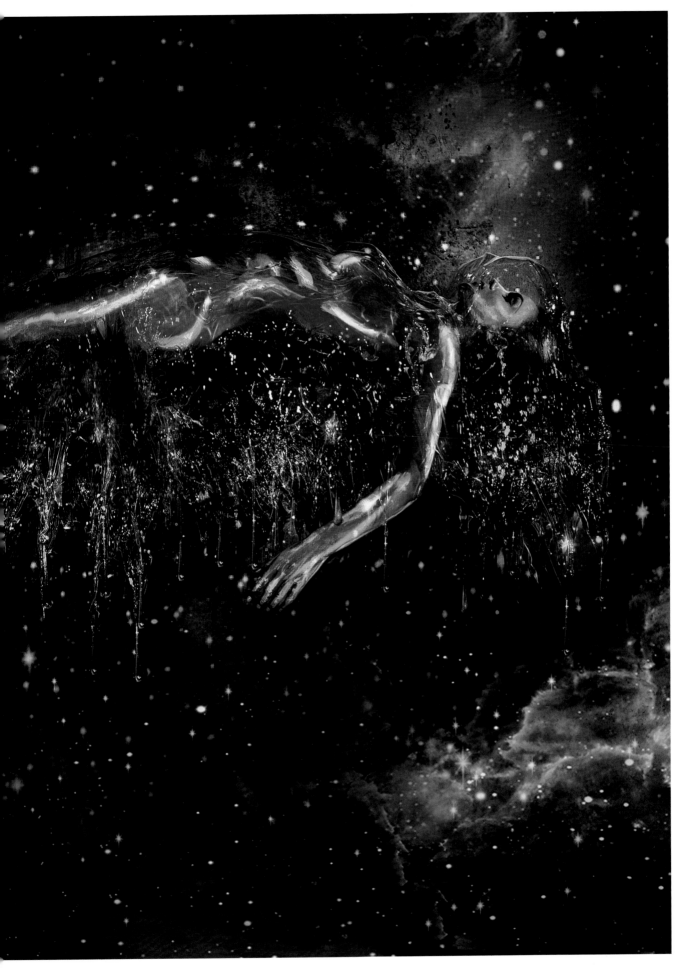

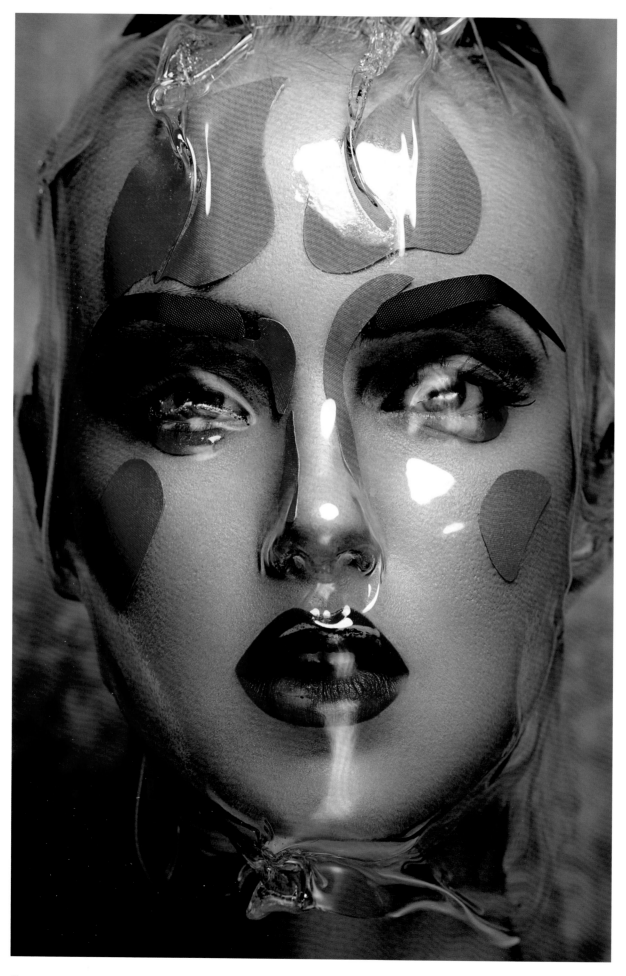

'The beauty industry relies on a desire to enhance reality. As digital technology advances, the gap between fantasy and reality expands. New expectations of more spectacular versions of ourselves will create the need for minimum effort with maximum-results products.'
– Phyllis Cohen, Makeup Artist

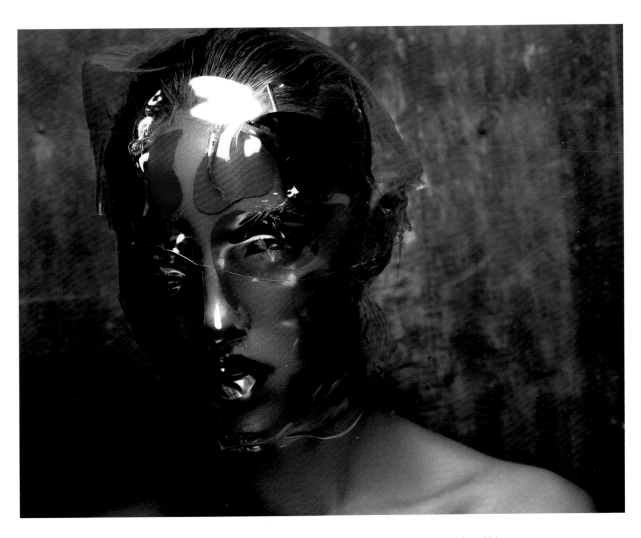

Pages 92-95 **Makeup** Kryolan Aquacolor 509; Make Up For Ever 12 Flash Color Case; NYX Studio Liquid Liner, Extreme Blue; Face•Lace **Photography** Camille Sanson **Hair** Diana Moar **Headpiece and Bodypiece** Justin Smith **Model** Karina @ Select **Makeup Assistant** Kerry White **Photography Assistant/Set Design** Rua Acorn, Lianna Fouler and Brendan Grealis

Pages 96-97 **Makeup** MAC Studio Face and Body Foundation, Lipstick (Ruby Woo), Eye Kohl (Smolder), Fluidline (Blacktrack), Strobe Cream, Chromagraph Pencil (Pure White), Eye Shadow (White Frost), Sculpting Powder Pro Palette (Shadester), Eye Brows, Liquid Eye Liner (Boot Black), Eylure lashes **Photography** Camille Sanson **Styling** Karl Willett **Clothes** (left to right) 1. jacket and hat (Atsuko Kudo), skirt (William Wilde), shoes (Vivian Ying); 2. dress (Chic Freak), gloves (KTZ), shoes (Kandee Shoes); 3. shirt (Sasha Louise),

lingerie (Agent Provocateur), boots (Vivian Ying); 4. shirt and trousers (Atsuko Kudo), shoes (Natacha Marro); 5. body (Atsuko Kudo), shoes (Natacha Marro); 6. lingerie (William Wilde), crop top, skirt and socks (Sasha Louise), headpiece (Jay Briggs), shoes (Natacha Marro) **Hair** Diana Moar **Models** (left to right) Jay-Jay @ Leni's, Alessa @ Storm, Lidiia @ Leni's and Karina @ Select **Styling Assistant** Adele Pentland **Makeup Assistant** Kerry White **Photography Assistant/Set Design** Rua Acorn, Lianna Fouler and Brendan Grealis

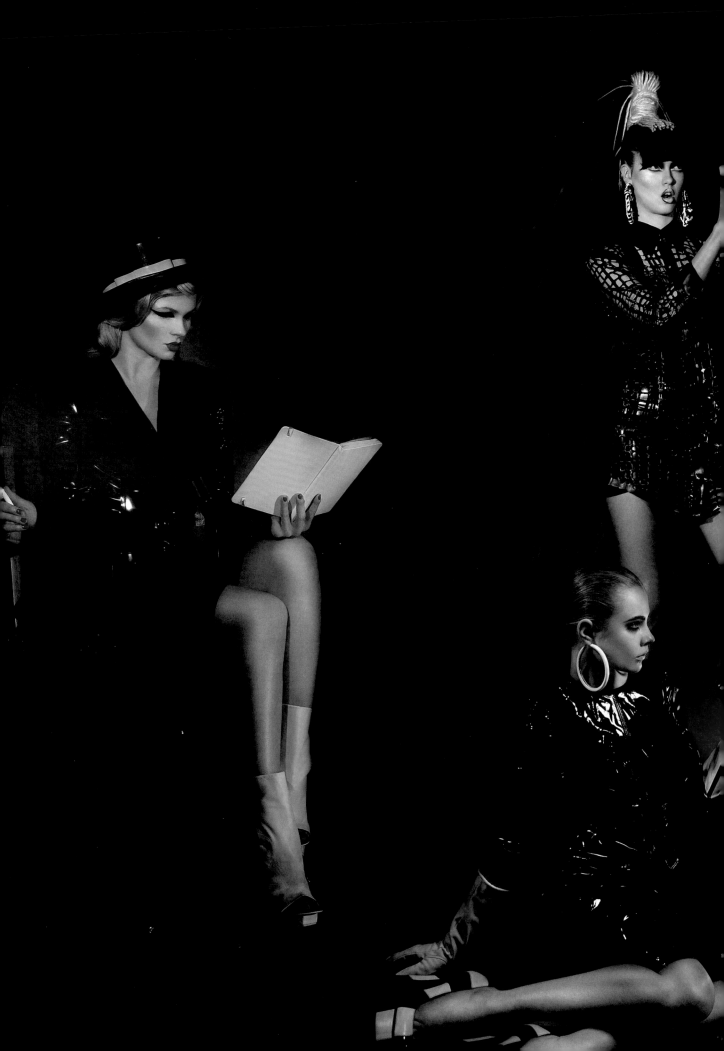

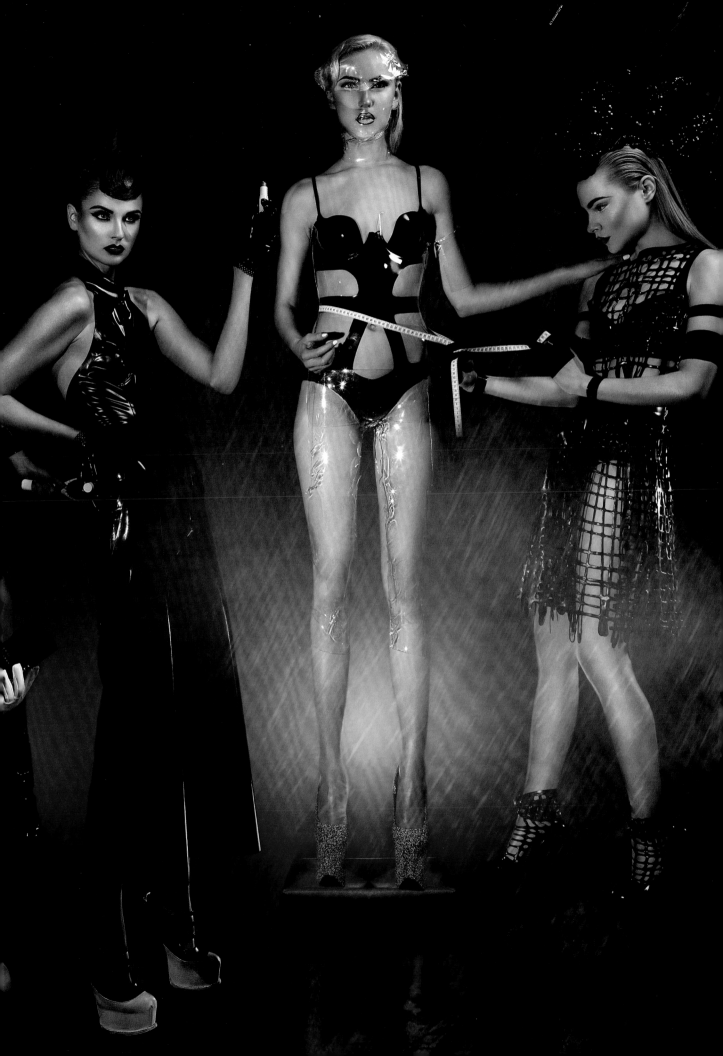

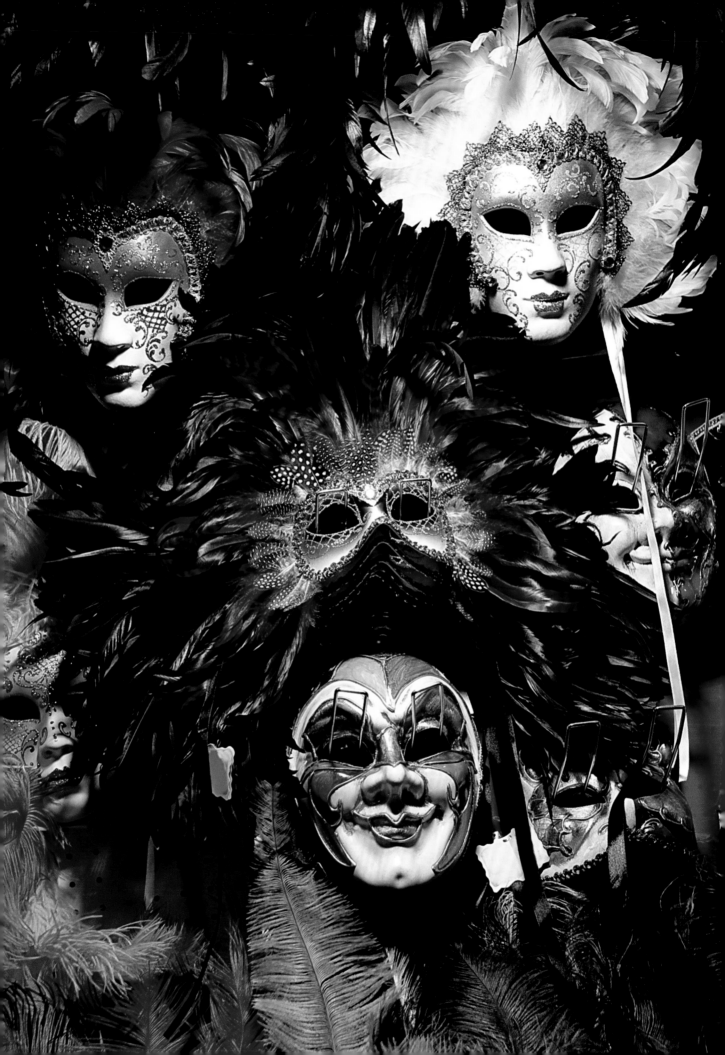

4. Performing Arts

The opera, the ballet, drag artists, the circus

'Makeup is a mask, and without it we cannot create character and expression to bring a performance to life.'

Right **Makeup** Kryolan TV Paint Stick (TV White), HD Cream Liner, Aquacolor Dayglow Palette; Eyelure Definition No 121 Lashes **Photography** Catherine Harbour **Hair** Chie Sato using Label.m **Model** Angela Hsu **Makeup Assistant** Yuko Fredrikkson

Below **Makeup** Kryolan Supracolor Greasepaint, Glitters **Photography** Catherine Harbour **Hair** Jose Quijano using Catwalk by TIGI **Styling and Dress** Joey Bevan, from his collection for the Queen's 2014 Coronation Festival **Model** Millie

The performing arts

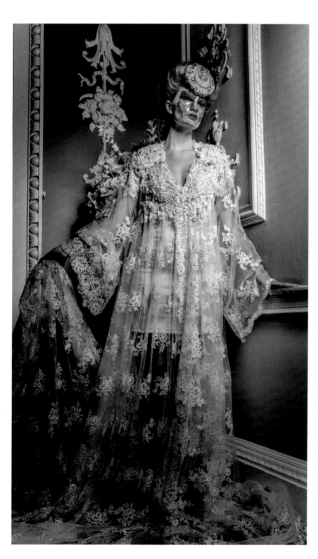

Creating specific characters is an essential part of being a creative makeup artist in performance – in worlds as diverse as the theatre, dance, ballet, opera and circus. Often, actors will have to apply their own makeup due to time or budget constraints, so this section is dedicated to creating some looks that can be tailored for different themes, but are ultimately fun! Makeup for performing arts is designed to exaggerate features as the audience is far away, and from Roman to Renaissance times crude face paint consisted of white powder, chalk, burnt cork and mineral pigments. Early stage lighting consisted of candles, and later gas lamps, which were forgiving when it came to the crudeness of the application. With the invention of electricity came harsher production lighting, simultaneously showing every flaw while bleaching out the facial features. Greasepaint was invented in the 1860s in Germany by Ludwig Leichner, a Wagnerian opera singer, and was originally formulated simply from pigment and lard. It's still one of my favourite mediums to use today; versatile, quick to apply, with a long-lasting cream base. Pancake makeup was invented by Max Factor in 1914 – it's a water-based makeup that provides thick, matt coverage. The formulas have continued to evolve and today the ingredients are safer for the skin (early makeup even used toxic lead), and are designed to stay put for hours under hot stage lights. Formulas that are easier to apply allow actors more time to be creative.

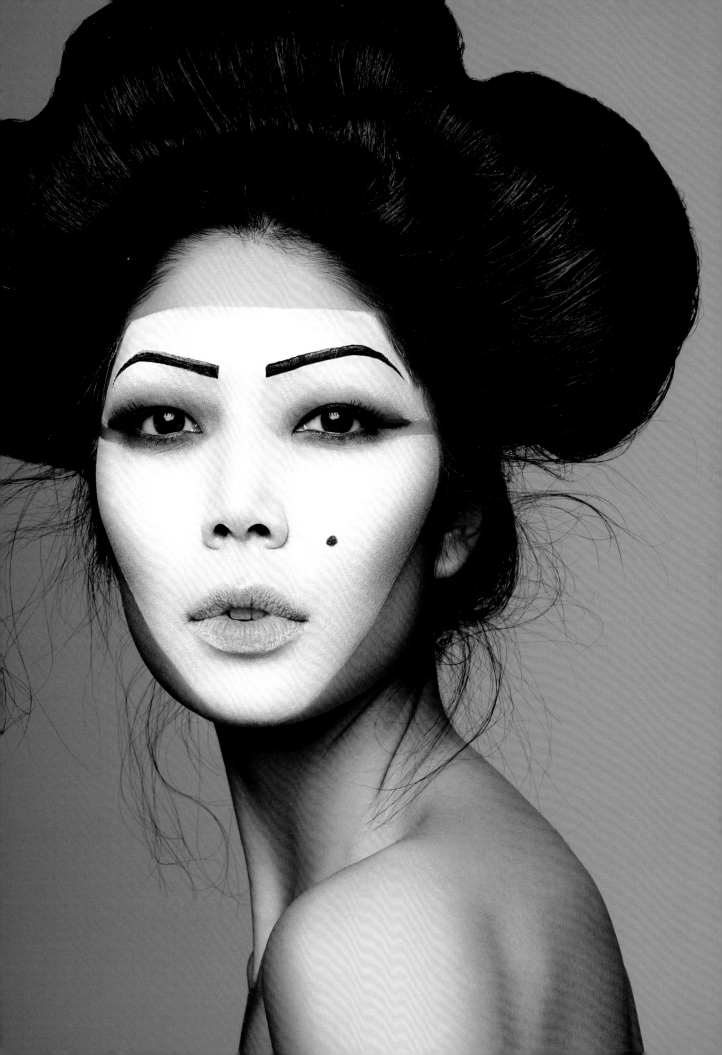

'Opera makeups were originally based on pale faces with exaggerated eyes, opulent and dramatic.'

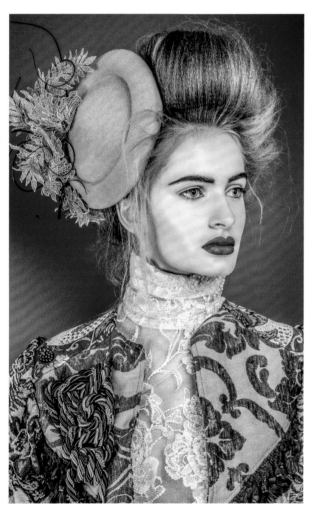

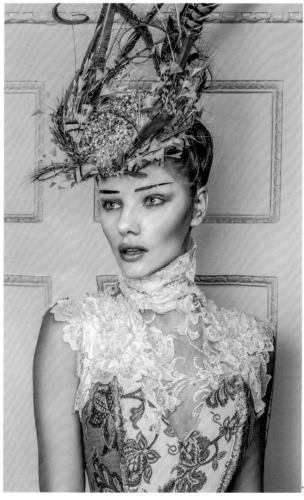

Above **Makeup** Bourjois Rouge Edition Velvet
(06, Pink Pong), Sourcil brow pencil, Intense
Eye Shadow (09) **Model** Millie

Right **Makeup** Kryolan Glamour Glow
Palette, Cine-Wax, Spirit Gum; MAC Studio
Face and Body Foundation (White), Paint Pot
(Constructivist), Lip Pencil (Subculture)
Model Myra

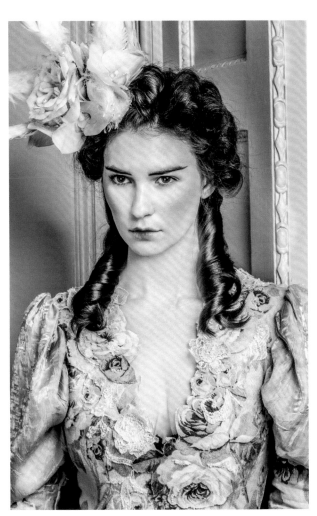

The opera

Traditional opera makeup was all about making the features much bigger and simple, with bold colours. Lots of lashes and bright colours that lasted well under stage lights was the key. Sometimes dramatic face masks were used instead, so all that was needed was a statement lip and wig to create the character. The Chinese Opera is particularly interesting, with its different stylized facial expressions symbolizing a character's personality, role and fate. For example, a red face represents loyalty and bravery, a black face – valour, yellow and white faces – duplicity, while golden and silver faces invoke mystery. Another example of this type of makeup is that of the geisha, the traditional Japanese female entertainer who acts as a hostess and whose skills include performing various Japanese arts. Traditionally the main process was to layer a thick paste of white foundation over the face and neck, removing the eyebrows and painting a false eyebrow high on the forehead in thick black paint. Eyes had a hint of red and black, which would decrease as they matured, finished with small red lips painted in the centre of their natural shape. This lengthy and skilled process continues to influence fashion editorial makeup today.

Makeup Kyrolan TV Paint Stick (TV White), HD Cream Liner (Ebony), Eye Shadow Variety Palette; The Body Shop Lip and Cheek Stain
Model Hannah

All: **Photography** Catherine Harbour **Hair** Jose Quijano using Catwalk by TIGI **Styling** Joey Bevan and the collection he designed for the Queen's 2014 Coronation Festival

'Makeup is always defined and heavy
to bring out our features on stage.'
– *Amber Doyle, Ballerina*

The ballet

If you think of the ballet, what often springs to mind is *Swan Lake*, with the iridescent skin, black eyeliner and pale lips of the white swan princess, Odette, and the vampish, elongated eyes with silvers and blacks of the black swan, Odile. Two contrasting characters, the good swan and the bad swan, who are equally haunting and beautiful on stage.

Dancer Amber Doyle explains, 'Classical ballet dancers like me always do our own stage makeup. Often we have a week of lessons to help us learn to do our makeup to the style of the show. With help from professional makeup artists we are then able to recreate the same look every night, which can involve having three different makeup changes for every act. We always use a thick foundation, and thick eyeliner to define the eyes.

'Eyelashes are usually black and thick to be seen on the stage, and cheekbones heavily shaded. I often use white on the lid before going into the eye socket with a dark grey or black, and lines are also often put under the eye to add definition. When playing a character you often wear a more flamboyant style with coloured eyelashes, over-the-top lips, red rosy cheeks. But for classical dance the lashes are always black. For certain ballets you may also use more of a white base to give a ghostly appearance.'

Pages 105-109
Makeup Kryolan Shimmery Skin Foundation Pearl, Kryolan Makeup Blend HD Micro Foundation Daniel Sandler watercolour fluid blusher cherub, Lip Emphasizer, Lip Rouge Sheer Palette 18 Colors **Photography** Camille Sanson **Stylist** Karl Willett **Hair** Diana Moar **Model** Deimante Misiunaite, Storm **Stylist's Assistants** Vivian Nwonka

Opposite page
Corset and skirt Giles **Shoes** Capezio

Page 106
Dress Jay Briggs **Shoes** Capezio

Page 107
Makeup as above with Shu Uemura False Feather lashes **Nails** Essie Blanc **Body** Jay Briggs **Cap** Atsuko Kudo

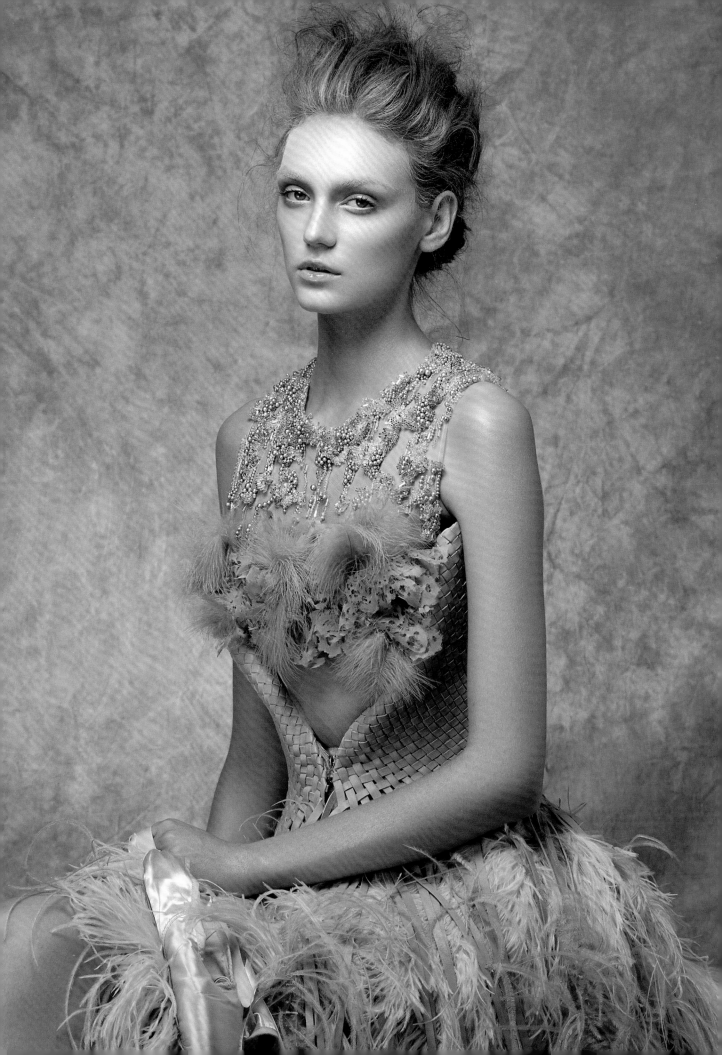

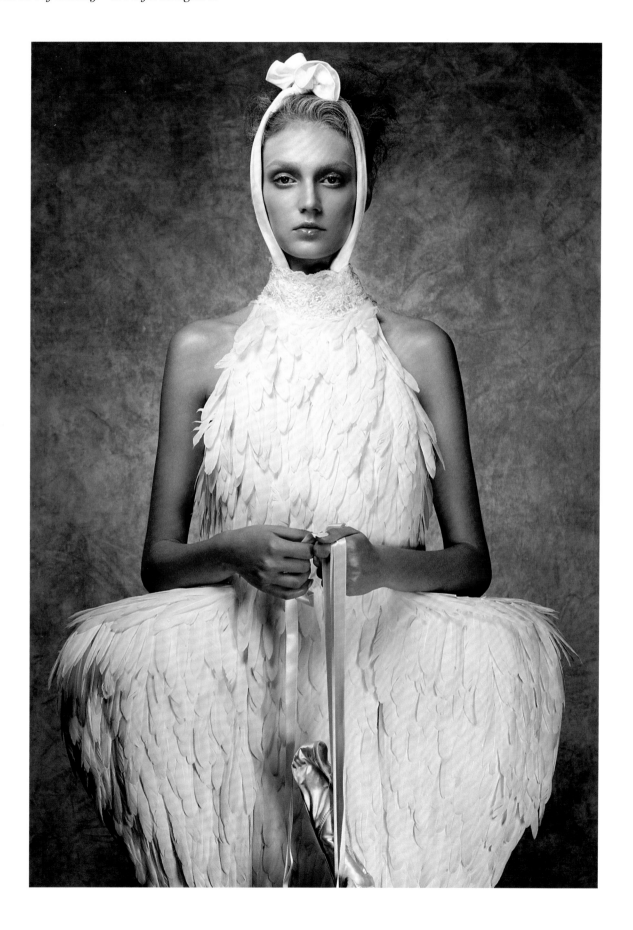

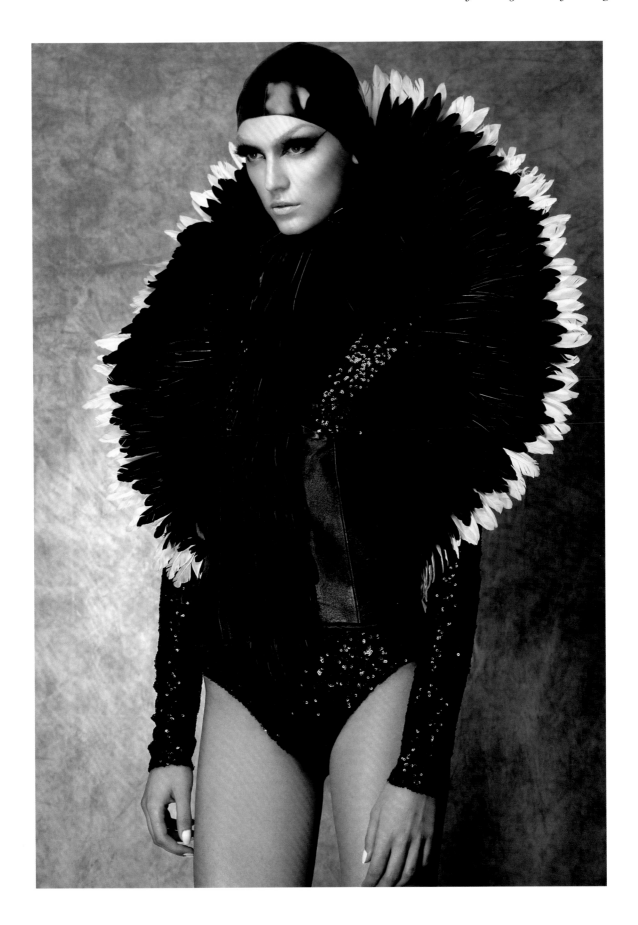

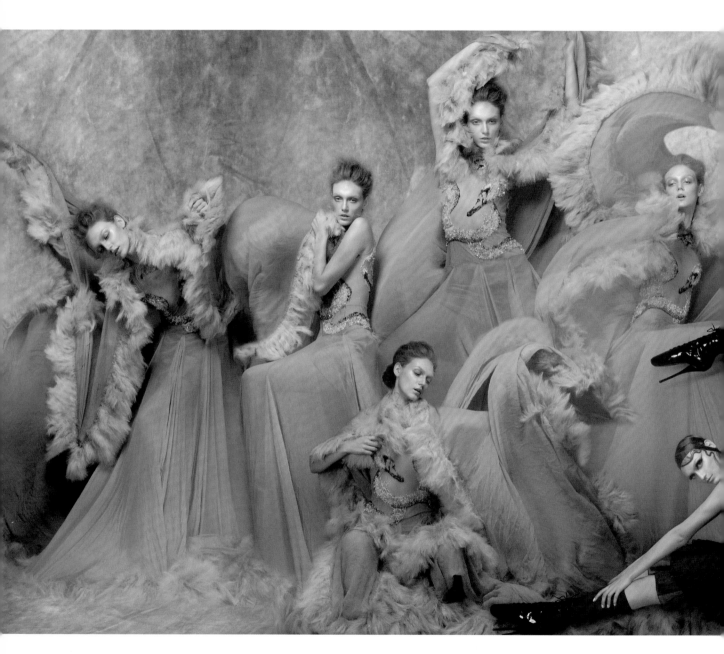

White dress Giles **Black corset and skirt**
Sorapol **Black cap and shoes** Atsuko Kudo

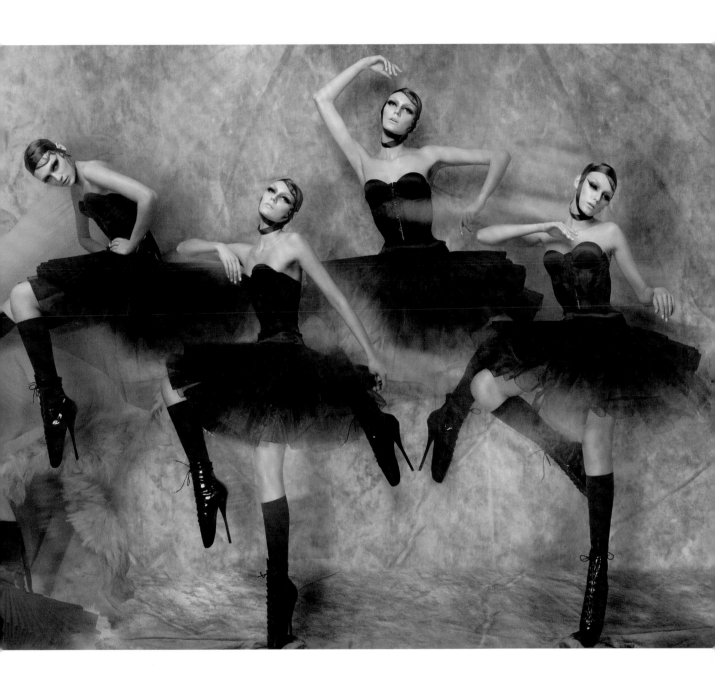

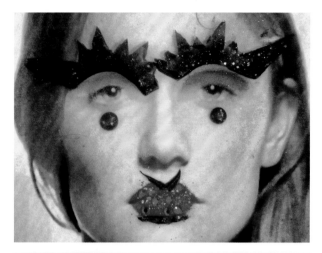

Top Lan's smudge chart

Left Photography Gary Nunn **Hair** Klare Wilkinson **Styling** Joey Bevan **Clothes** Ivanna Pila, sponsored by Kryolan at United Makeup Artists Expo 2013, London **Headpiece** Louis Mariette

Right Photography Gary Nunn **Styling** Joey Bevan **Clothes** Inbar Spector, sponsored by Kryolan, shot at the Royal Opera House **Model** Imogen Leaver

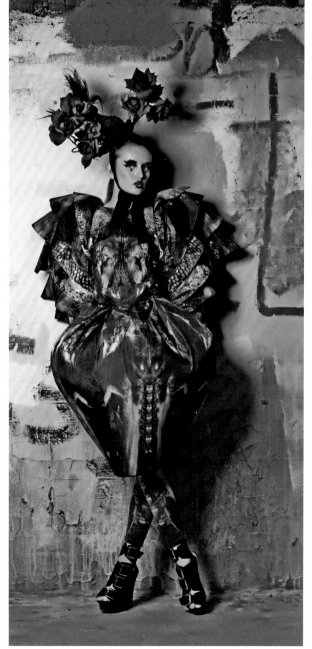

Drag artists

Drag makeup works on enhancing beauty and exaggerating the features to make them more feminine. All masculine features are first blanked out, then worked back in again to female perfection. Everything is flawless and cleanly done, and there is a lot to be learnt from the drag artist's application techniques, where more is more. The Fabulous Russella, London's darling of drag, explains:

'I generally tend to be a blonde so I pull inspiration from other blondes such as Jayne Mansfield or Marilyn Monroe, who actually had very simple makeup, a red lip and mostly nude eye. I used to sit and copy other drag queens as they were doing their makeup in the mirror. Eventually I came to "find my face" and I know what suits me now. I always wear a glitter lip, which has become a bit of a signature look now. As a guy my lips are fairly thin and I'm not a huge fan of going over the lip line with lipstick unless it's done exceptionally well, so covering my mouth in red glitter hides the fact that my lips are thin. As I lip-synch it's important that my lips stand out, so glittering them makes them sparkle in the stage lights and draws focus. However, I also love a smoky eye – the Kardashians seem to have the smoky eye well executed. I was once taught by another drag queen that if I can perfect the eye it doesn't matter how messy my lip is – I don't know how true this is, but I can pull off a messy lip, but never a messy eye.'

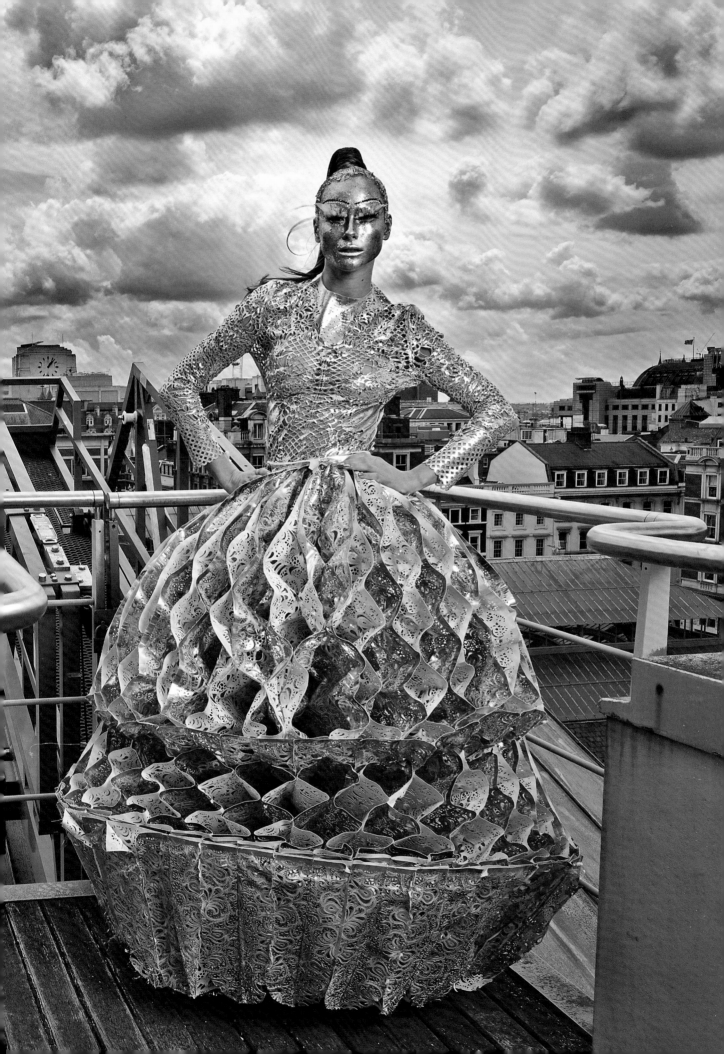

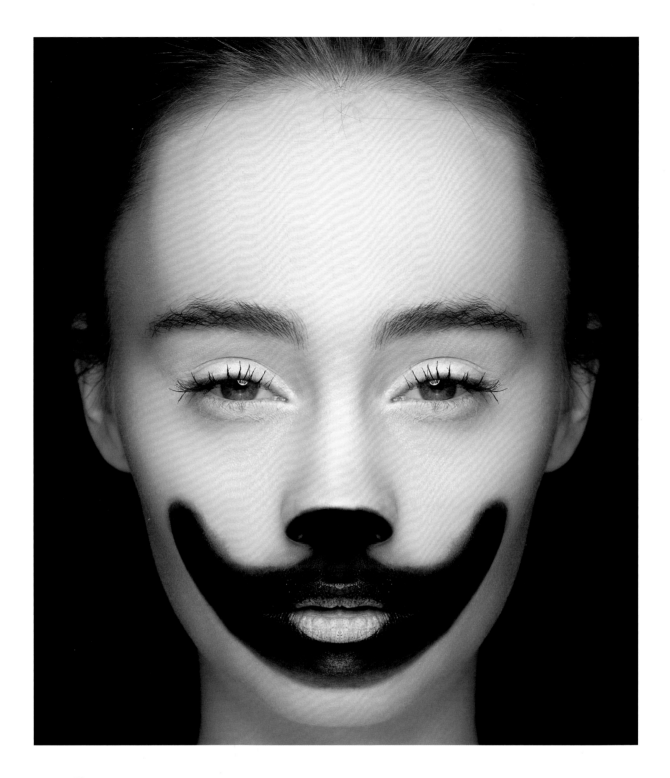

The circus

Some of my favourite productions are those staged by Cirque du Soleil, for the outrageous and complex makeup styles that they have for each character. I remember heading to the circus as a young girl and seeing the clowns, with their white face makeup, and either sad faces or mischievous grins with red lips stretched widely across their faces – some were quite scary! While traditional clowns have exaggerated

wigs, footwear, shapes painted on their cheeks and, invariably, a red nose, for a fashion editorial I created a pared-down version, with the white face paint thinned out to look more porcelain, and only washes of colour. Details around the eyes, like a teardrop or simple line that fades to the centre of the face, are more simplified and graphic, or you can just work on a statement big lip in different colours.

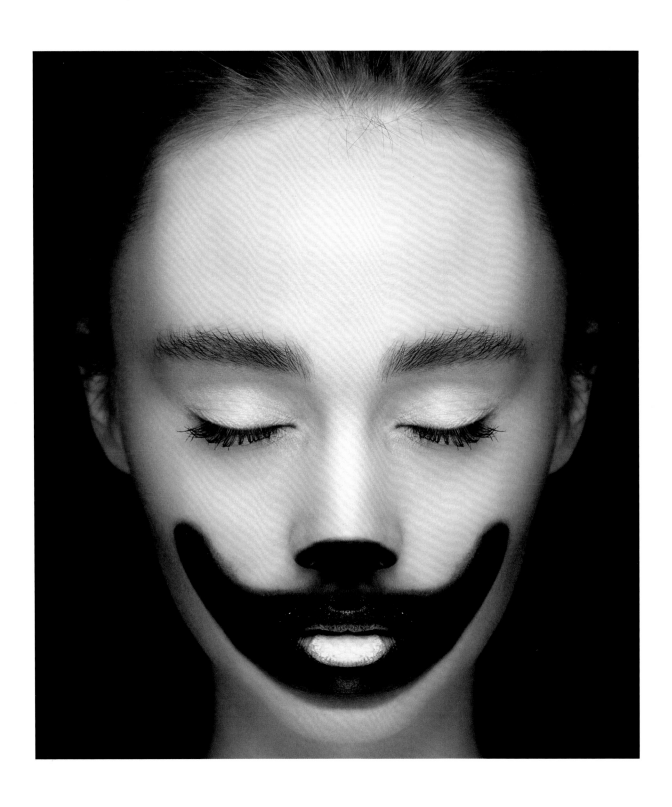

Makeup MAC Studio Face and Body
Foundation (White), Full Coverage Foundation
(White), Chromagraph Pencil (Pure White),
Eye Shadow (White Frost, Bio Green),
Extended Play Gigablack Lash, Grease Paint
stick, Pigment (Teal) **Photography** Catherine
Harbour **Model** Rae Matthews @ Nevs

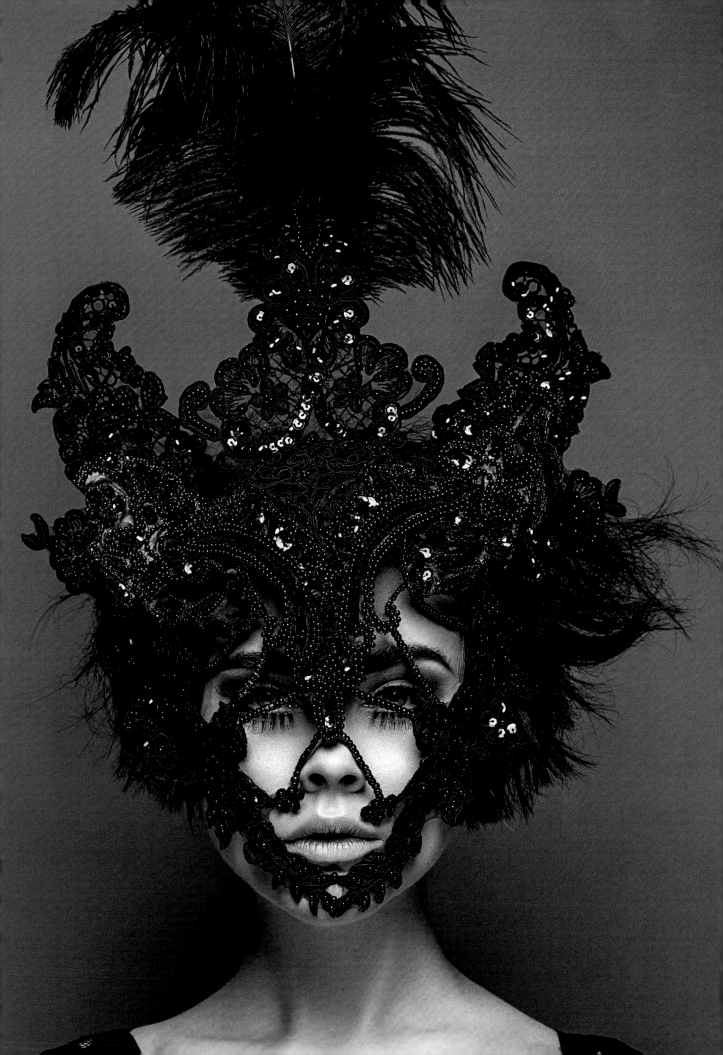

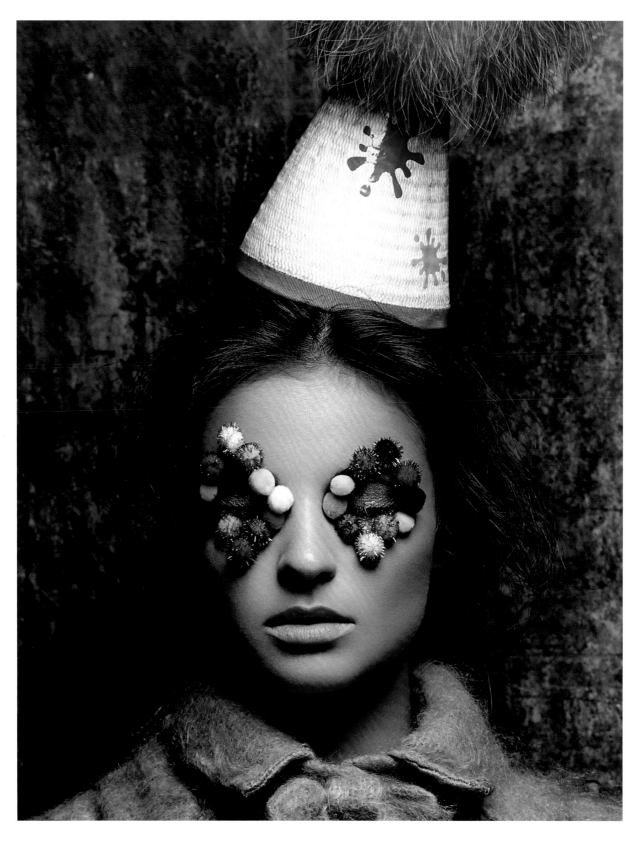

Left **Makeup** MAC Mineralize Foundation
NC15, Liquid Eye Liner (Boot Black), Eye
Shadow (Carbon), Lip Erase, Lashes
Photography Camille Sanson **Hair** Diana
Moar **Styling** Karl Willett **Headpiece** Jay
Briggs **Model** Lidiia @ Leni's

Above **Makeup** Kryolan Supracolor
Palette 24 Colors N **Photography** Camille
Sanson **Hair** Diana Moar using Bumble
and Bumble **Styling** Karl Willett **Jacket**
Christian Cowan-Sanluis **Hat** Piers
Atkinson **Model** Alessa @ Storm

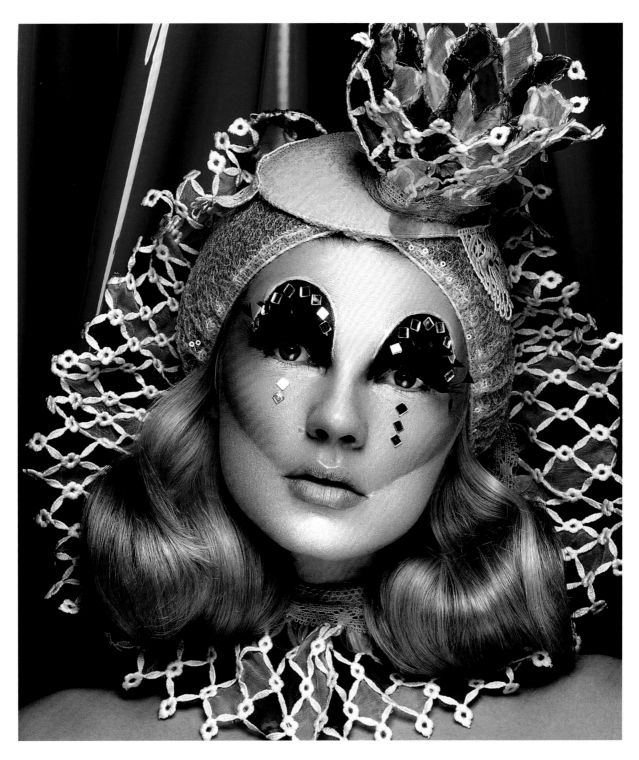

Manipulating highlights and shadows is so important for changing the face of any character in stage work as features are more pronounced under the stage lights. Highlights are used on the bridge of the nose, under the eyes, cheekbones and just below the brows. Using shades that are deeper than the skin tone provides depth and definition, most commonly used in the sockets, to thin the side of the nose, to sallow the cheeks and minimize heaviness under the chin. This technique is often used to age a character.

The eyes and brows are the most expressive features, so are very important for an actor. Eyeliner is essential for definition, to frame the eyes on top and bottom. Plenty of mascara is used on the top and bottom layer, with powder pressed in to thicken the lashes. A generous amount of powder is important to set the makeup and avoid shine.

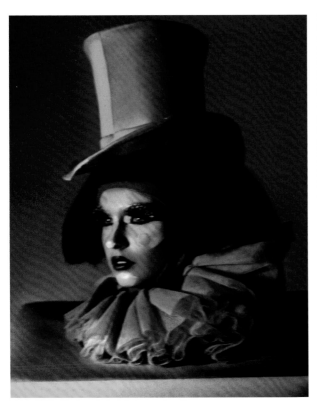

Left **Makeup** Kryolan Aquacolor
UV-Dayglow, Supracolor Shimmering
Vision Palette, Kajal Pencil, HD Cream
Liner, Lipstick Classics (LC007, LC102);
Shu Uemura eyelashes **Photography**
Camille Sanson **Hair** Diana Moar
Styling Karl Willett **Hat and Neckpiece**
National Theatre Costume **Model**
Alessa **Makeup Assistant** Kerry White

Far left **Makeup** Bourjois Smoky Stories
Palette (07, In Mauve), Blush (34, Rose
d'Or), Intense Eyeshadows (03, 10),
Rouge Edition 12-hour lipstick (32,
Rose Vanity), Rouge Edition Velvet (01,
Personne ne rouge; 32), Effect 3D
Lipgloss (29, Rose Charismatic) **Clothes**
Justin Smith **Model** Jay Jay

Cirque du Soleil holds the title as the largest theatrical producer in the world, and to this day over 90 million people have seen their shows. Since 1995 Cirque's makeup designer Nathalie Gagné has crafted more than 1,000 separate makeup designs for 16 shows, including *Michael Jackson ONE*, as well as the 3D movie *Cirque du Soleil: Worlds Away*, produced by James Cameron. Nathalie was one of the first graduates of the Montreal branch of the famed Paris-based makeup school, the Christian Chauveau École de macquillage.

What inspires the make-up looks for the live shows?
'Anything can inspire me really, whether it is insects or architecture. Everything starts from the story I tell myself because every makeup design has its own story, which I then tell to the performers when I teach them how to reproduce the makeup (at Cirque du Soleil, performers are responsible for putting on their own makeup). I find it is easier for the performer to be told a makeup design story rather than to have some lines imposed on to his or her face. The performer develops a better sense of ownership with the makeup design this way.'

How does the makeup add to the overall costume effect?
'The makeup completes the costume. It is fused to the face and body. It carries the emotion and is the magic final touch that transforms an acrobat into

character. The makeup is the soul of the character. Costume and makeup need each other to serve the character.'

What are some of the challenges creating makeup looks for performance?
'Performers perspire a lot and I always have to think about that when designing makeup for a show. Their performance is very demanding and the makeup should not be an obstacle to it. Performers should feel comfortable when wearing their makeup. My goal is to create makeups that will remain beautiful, even on a two-show night. Sometimes, a performer will play more than one character and my challenge will be to create a hybrid makeup or one that will be easy to adapt for each of his or her characters.'

Do you have any tricks and tips when it comes to creating makeup looks for the performing arts?
'It is very important to respect the shape of the face and its muscles in order to have a makeup that will live and express emotions, otherwise the makeup becomes merely a mask.'

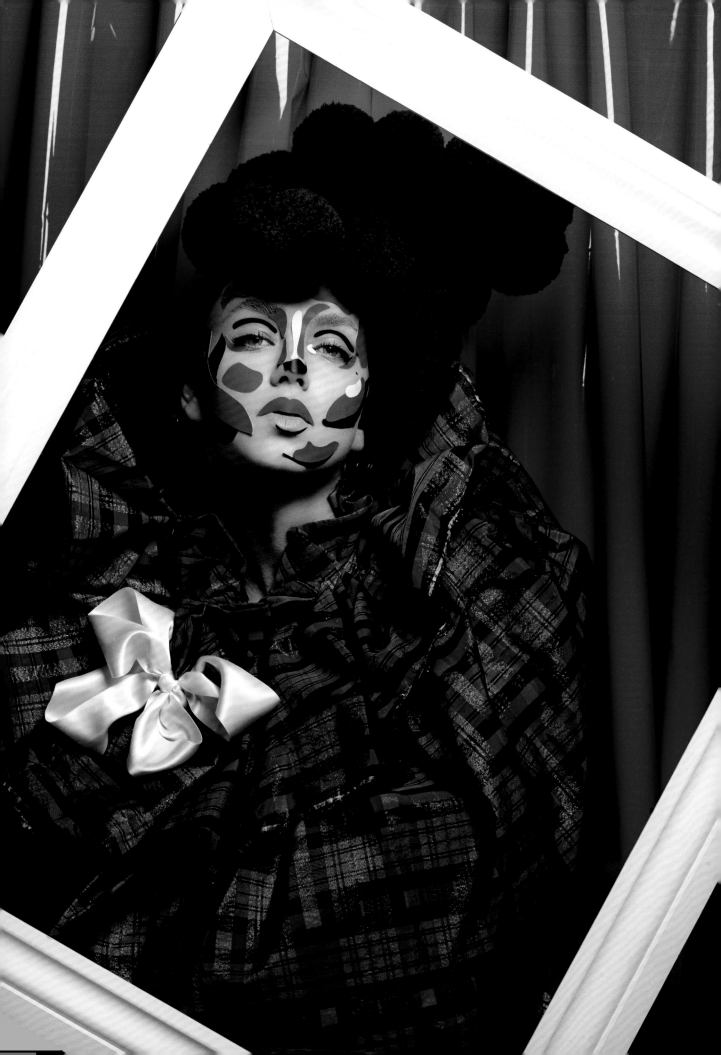

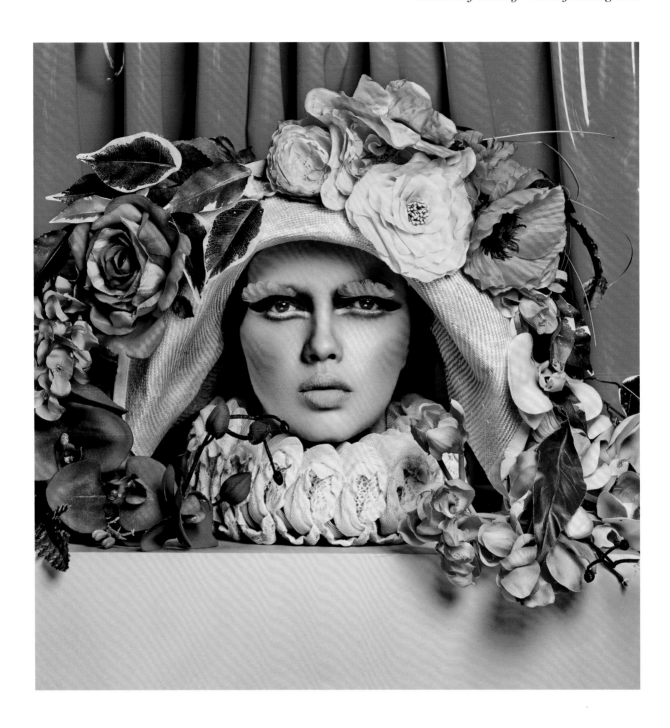

Left **Makeup** MAC Studio Face and Body
Foundation (White), Full Coverage Foundation
(W10), Lipglass, Penultimate Eye Liner, Zoom
Lash; Face•Lace **Cape** Sorapol **Hat** Justin Smith
Model Karina White @ Select

Above **Makeup** Kryolan Variety Palette (V1,
Pearl), Paint Stick (TV White), HD Cream
Liner, Eyelashes **Hat** Piers Atkinson **Model**
Alessa @ Storm

Team credits, both: **Photography** Camille Sanson
Hair Diana Moar **Styling** Karl Willett **Makeup
Assistant** Kerry White **Styling Assistant** Adele
Pentland

The A

Busi

Art of
ness

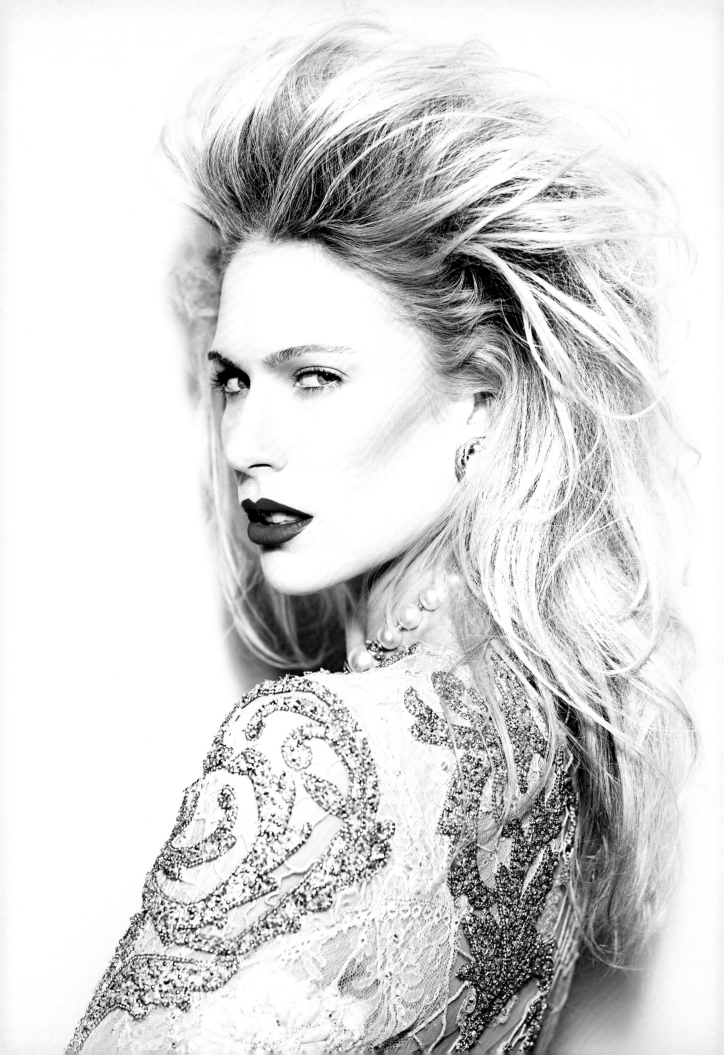

5. *Fashion and Editorial*

'*In this section I share various techniques and ideas for working in the industry, with an added artistic twist.*'

'*It was such an honour for me to be a part of this project. As a model, makeup is such an integral part of how you feel on a shoot. Working with Lan is always such a pleasure. She really understands how to work with a face and adapt her vision to suit your features.*'

– Tuuli, Model

Tuuli
by Rankin

One face and four looks was my theme in working with Rankin and his muse Tuuli. This shows how the transformation from one look to another is possible and almost extreme beyond recognition. Working from a blank canvas I first created a high-fashion simple statement look with a red lip; I changed her skin texture and added more contrast to turn her into a futuristic doll-like character with a super-shiny skin texture and fuller glossy lips with winged eyes. From there I built up the colours, also 'removing' her eyebrows to create a 1920s' couture goddess with purple and pink tones that exaggerated the features using glitter textures and shine. Working on top of this I then gave her a tribal look with multicoloured use of paint and textures in glitter and beading, which gave the face another dimension. Building up the layers Tuuli was immersed in vibrant colours. The final image is another extreme look that is a darker version, with stronger graphic colour tones and lines. By changing the styling completely she becomes almost like a creature from out of this world.

All images **Photography** Rankin **Hair** Klare Wilkinson using Kevin Murphy **Model** Tuuli **Hair Assistant** James Langan

Previous page **Makeup** Kryolan UV-Dayglow Compact Color Palette, HD Micro Foundation Palette; MAC Lip Pencil (Cherry), Lipsticks (Ruby Woo, Lady Danger) **Dress** Julien Macdonald **Jewellery** Liz Mendez Vintage

Opposite **Dress and Headpiece** Furne One

Following page **Makeup** Kryolan Supracolor Shimmering Vision Palette; MAC Chromagraph Pencil (Pure White), Full Coverage Foundation (W10), Studio Face and Body Foundation (White), Lipstick (Russian Red); Yves Saint Laurent Effet Faux Cils Shocking Eyeliner **Bodysuit** Hasan Hejazi

Page 126 **Makeup** Kryolan Supracolor Shimmering Vision Palette, Multi Gel Glitter, HD Cream Liners; MAC Eye Kohl (Smolder), Glitter (Red, Turquoise); Make Up For Ever 12 Flash Color Case; Ciaté beads **Cape** Nicolas Oakwell **Headpiece** Vicki Sarge

Page 127 **Jacket** Hasan Hejazi **Turban** Philip Treacy **Rings** Vicki Sarge **Necklaces** Liz Mendez Vintage

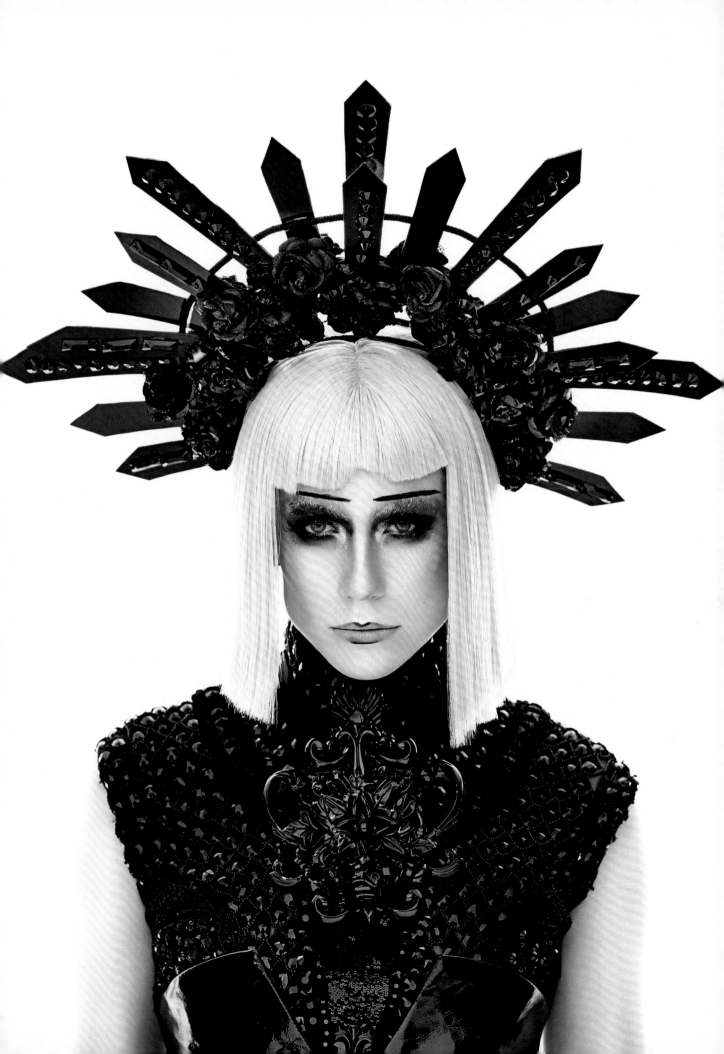

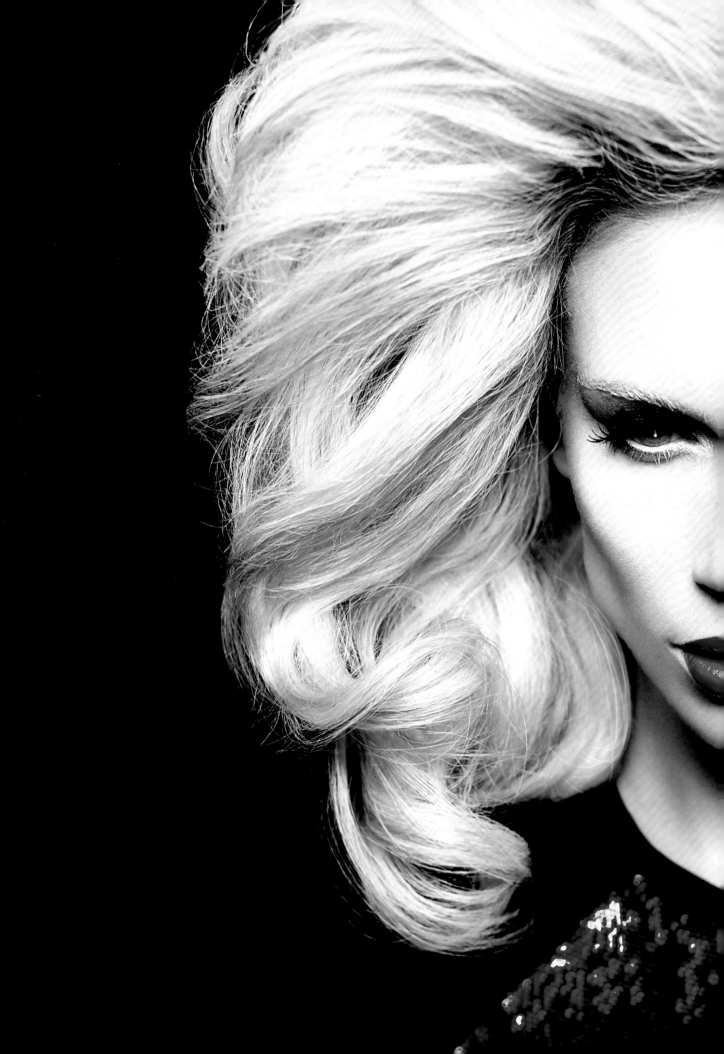

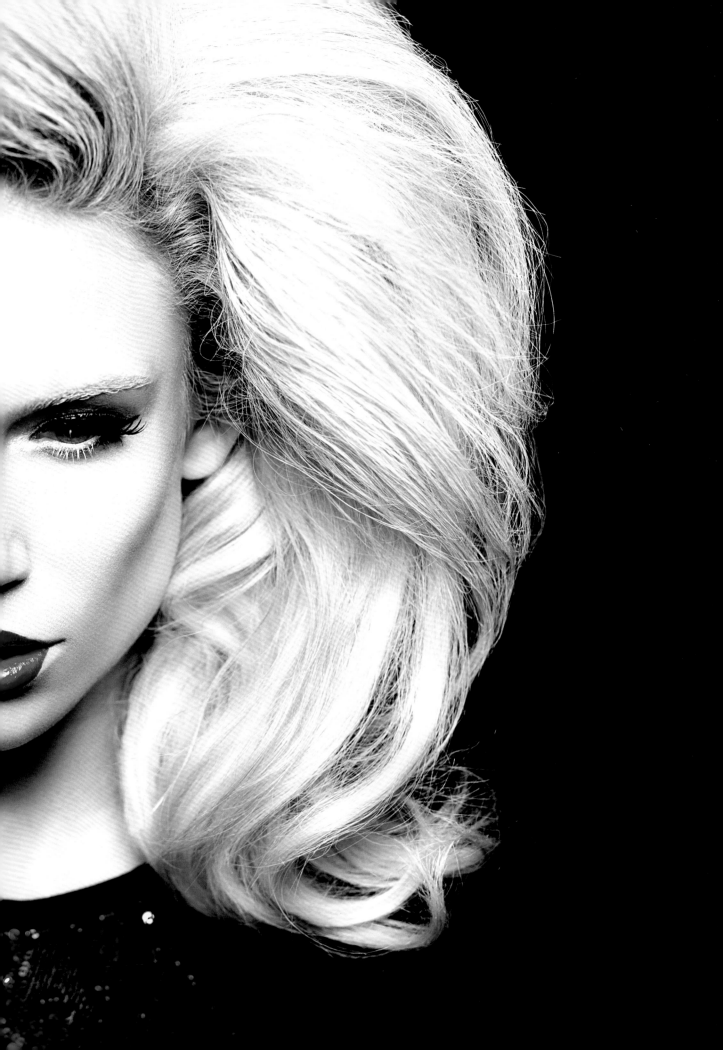

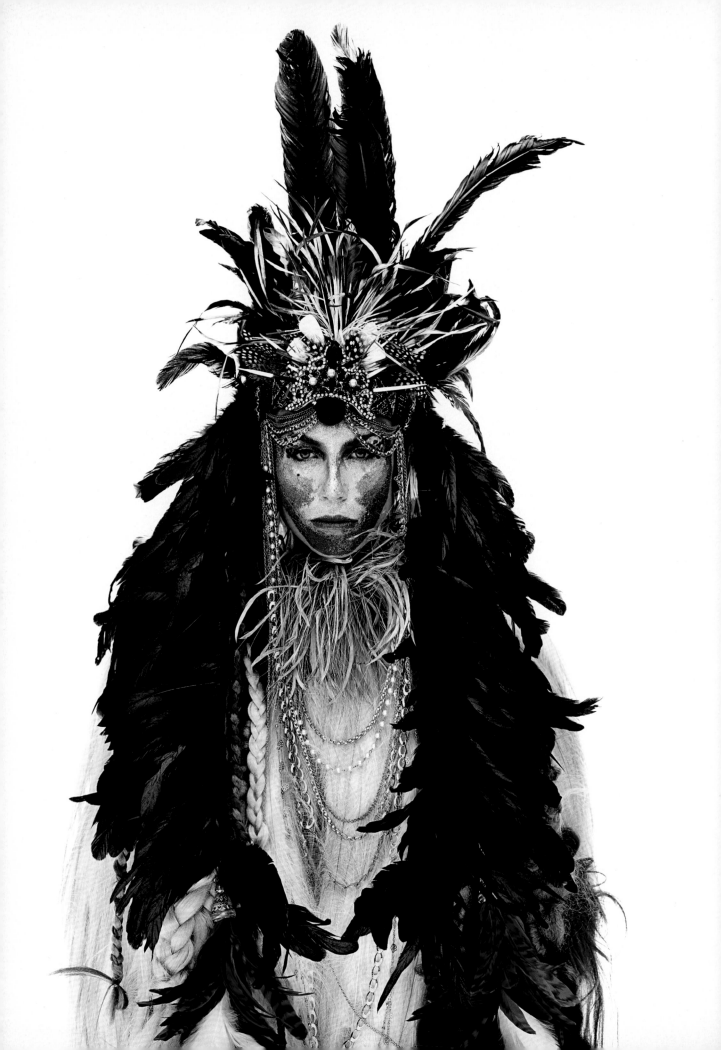

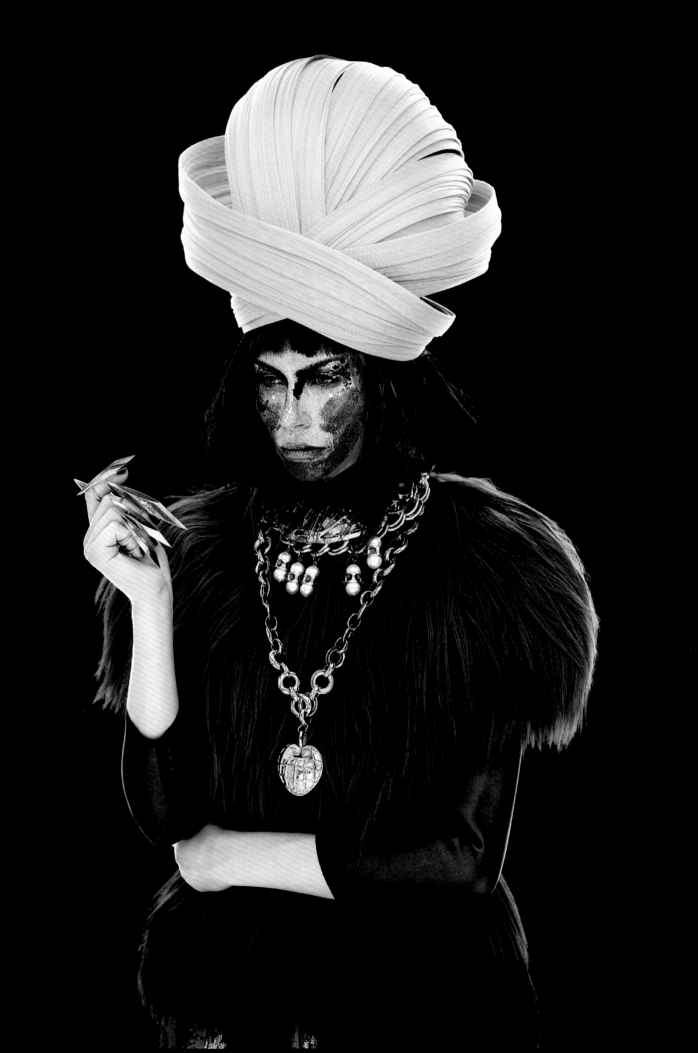

Creating beautiful images

I believe that beauty is in the eye of the beholder; everything you see in these pages is just my personal interpretation and ideas of how I see beauty, starting from a blank canvas. Using models' looks as a starting point I create an image that I feel displays art and beauty in its own way. Whether it is the hair design, the clothes, the headdress or the lighting of the finished image, as a whole it is all significant in showcasing the beauty. Working with the right photographer can bring the makeup to a different level, beyond your own imagination. The relationship between the photographer and artist is very significant as there is only so much retouching that can be relied upon.

At the beginning of my career I didn't know about retouching and worked with new photographers who shot with basic film cameras. I would always aim to make my work so flawless that no retouching was needed. It is so rewarding to look at a beauty image knowing that it doesn't need to be retouched, and this is due to the work of the makeup artist. I still believe in working like this today. When digital photography became popular with clients, I was still not aware of the possibilities of retouching, and only when I saw examples of before and after shots online was I shocked to see the difference between good and bad makeup artistry.

Retouching is quite an important tool for removing hairs, lumps and bumps that are quite difficult to get rid of unless the makeup is really caked on. Some photographers prefer not to have foundation on the skin, as it's easier to fix blemishes in post-production with real skin rather than with a thick layer of fake skin that becomes flat in the overall image. It's so important to keep the skin as true to reality as possible. After all, foundation was designed to give a flawless base, but if the model has great skin then just a bit of moisturiser, highlighter and concealer is enough.

Makeup The Body Shop Lightening Touch, All-In-One Instablur, Shimmer Waves, Divide and Multiply Mascara, Colour Crush Eye Shadow (01, Sugar Gaze), Love Gloss for Lips (Natural) **Photography** Camille Sanson **Headpiece** Justin Smith **Model** Leila @ Profile

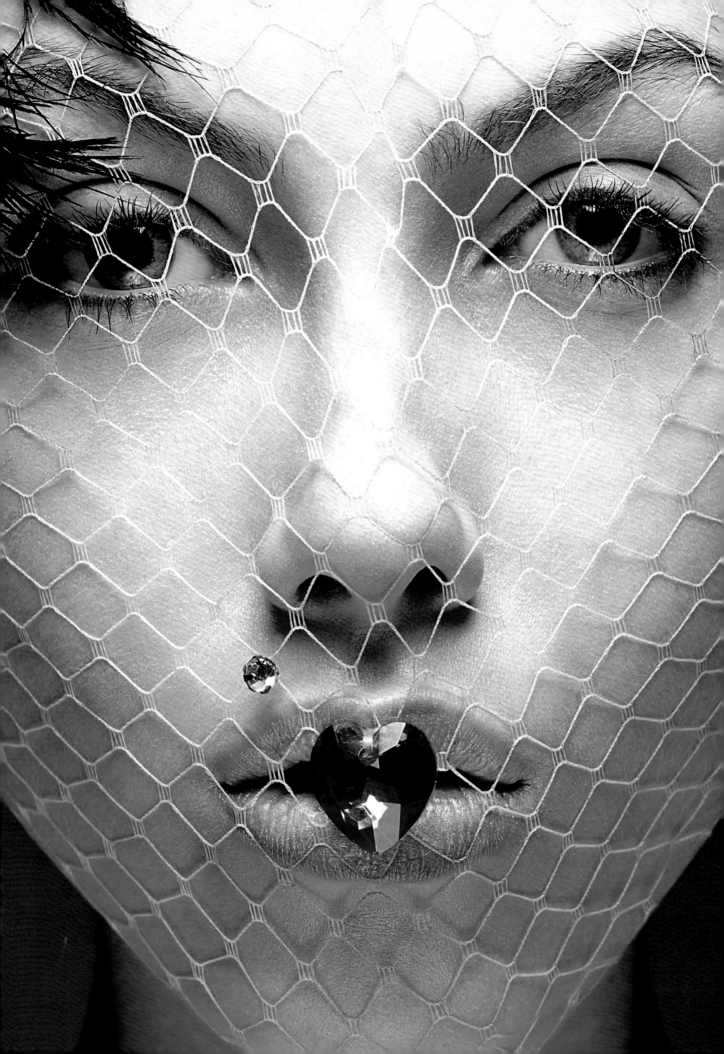

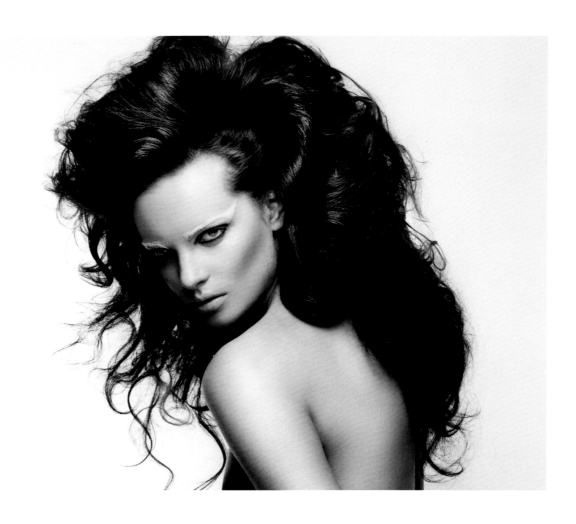

'*Like costume designers, makeup artists are storytellers. The relationship between hair stylists and makeup artists is a huge part of what brings any shoot to life. We do more than make models look good. We work closely with the rest of the team to bring the unimaginable to life.*'

– Diana Moar, Hair Stylist

Above **Makeup** Kryolan UV-Dayglow Compact Color Palette; MAC Chromagraph Pencil (Pure White), Eye Kohl (Smolder), Studio Face and Body Foundation, Sculpting Powder Pro Palette (Sculpt) **Photography** Camille Sanson **Hair** Diana Moar using Bumble and Bumble **Model** Mimi @ Premier

Opposite **Makeup** MAC Fluidline (Blacktrack), Lipglass on eyes, Lip Pencil (Redd), Lipstick (Russian Red), Strobe Cream **Photography** Camille Sanson **Hair** Diana Moar using Bumble and Bumble **Model** Barbara @ Leni's **Nails** Pebble Akins using Chanel

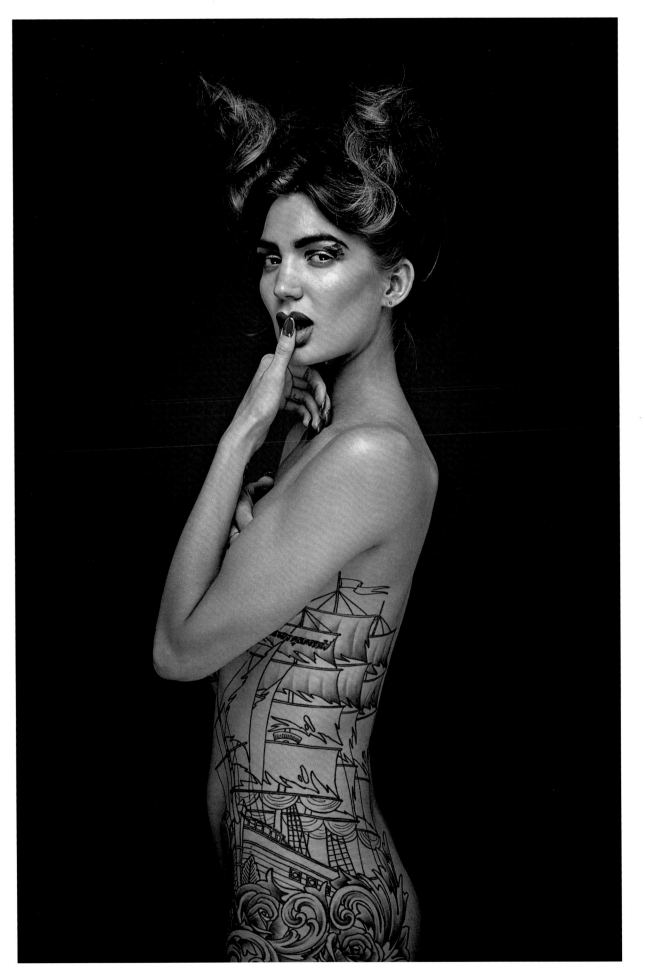

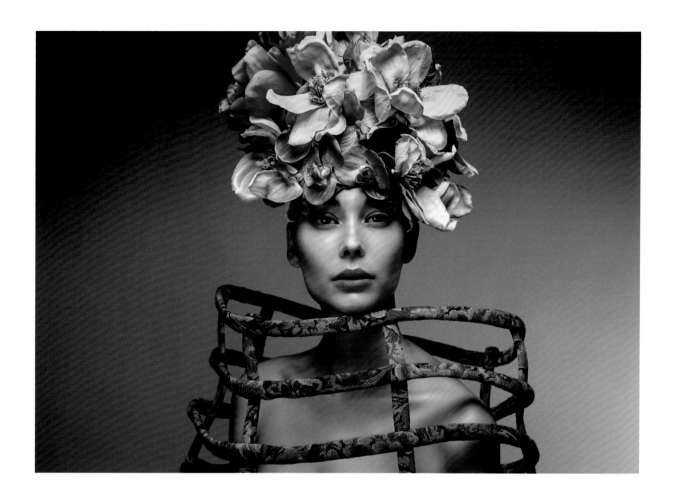

'A wise makeup artist once told me
that it isn't about the destination
but the journey. She was completely
right. Enjoy each step of your
career, as you grow and develop
as an artist.

Makeup The Body Shop Radiant Highlighter,
Touch of Light, Colour Crush Eye Shadow (001,
Sugar Gaze), Vitamin E Mist Spray, Colour
Crush Lipstick (101, Red Siren), Eyebrow 02
Kit **Photography** Camille Sanson **Hair** Diana
Moar **Styling** Karl Willett **Hat** MaryMe-Jimmy
Paul **Cage** William Tempest **Model** Joy @
Models 1

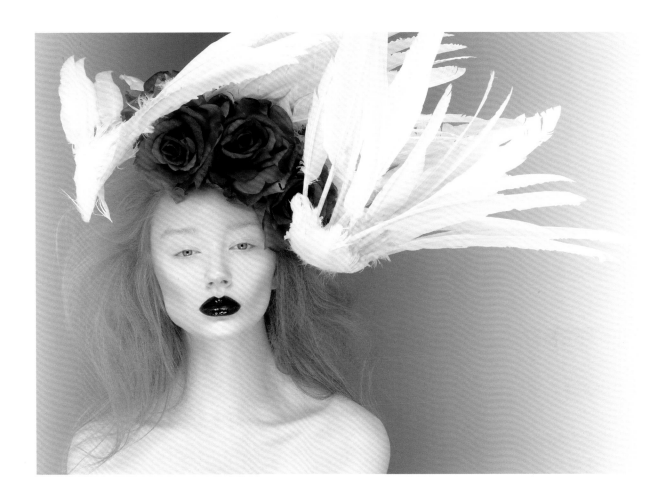

Never stop learning, seeking inspiration and, importantly, never compare your career to anyone else's! Ultimately, everyone has their own unique path.'

– Sandra Cooke, Makeup Artist

Makeup Kryolan TV Paint Stick (TV White);
MAC Studio Face and Body Foundation
(White), Studio Moisture Tint, Lip Pencil
(Burgandy); Yves Saint Laurent Rouge Pur
Couture Vernis à Lèvres Glossy Stain (Brun
Glace) **Photography** Camille Sanson **Hair**
Diana Moar **Styling** Karl Willett **Hat** Louis
Mariette **Model** Claudia D @ Premier

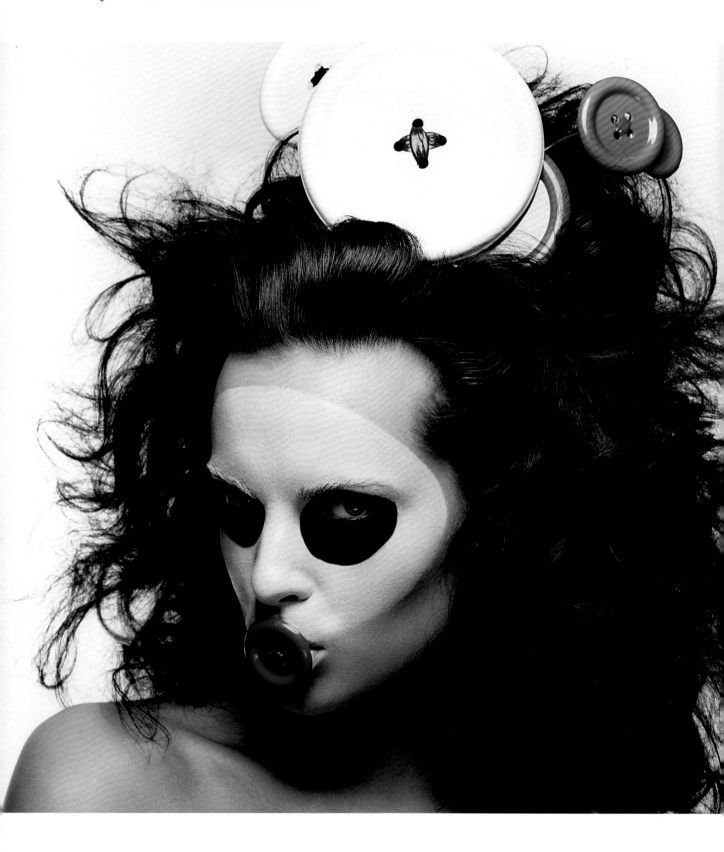

Makeup MAC Full Coverage Foundation
(White), Eye Kohl (Smolder), Fluidline
(Blacktrack), Grease Paint Stick **Photography**
Camille Sanson **Hair** Diana Moar using
L'Oreal Professional **Button Headpiece** Justin
Smith **Model** Barbara @ Leni's

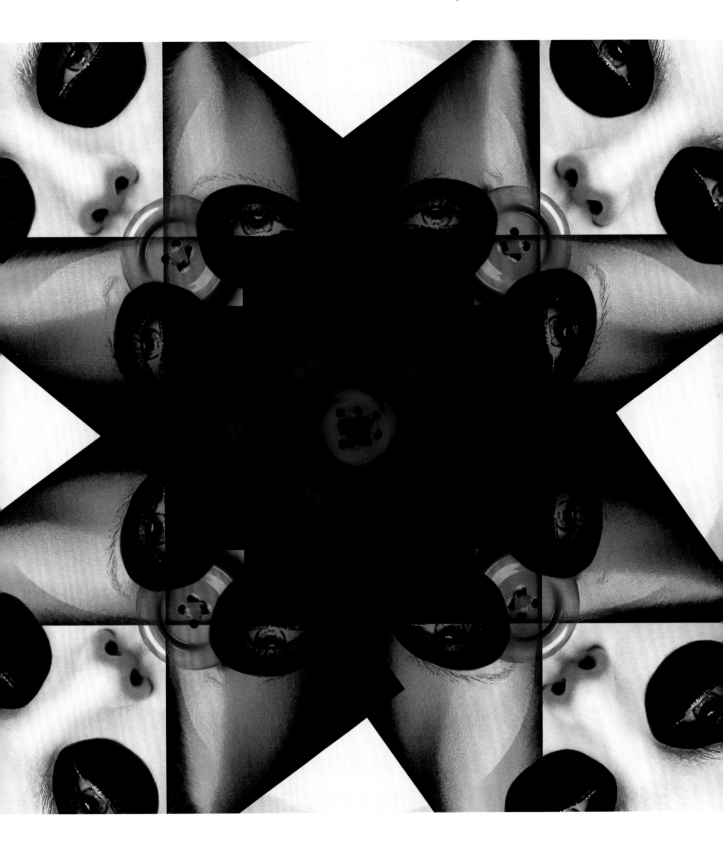

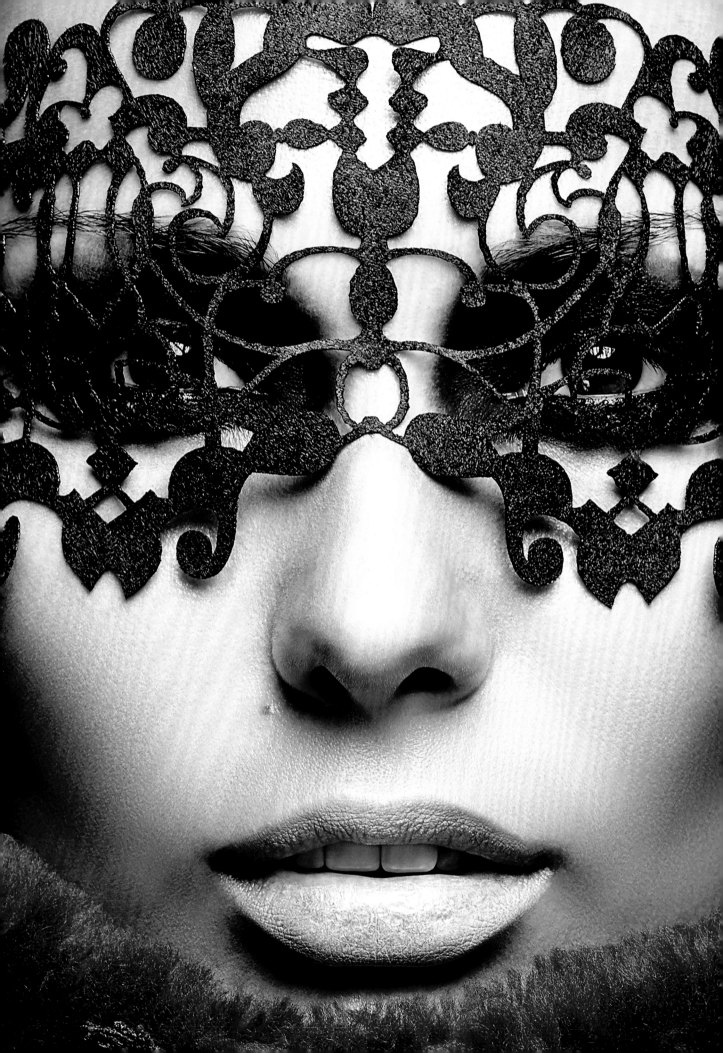

'Along with hair and wardrobe stylists, makeup artists are an essential part of the creative team. The industry has changed so much; it is no longer about somebody simply applying product, but rather creating a client's visual story and experience through the use of makeup.'

– Sacha Mascolo-Tarbuck,
Global Creative Director, Toni&Guy

Editorial

Editorial makeup, creating looks for the glossy magazines and advertising campaigns where the makeup doesn't distract attention from clothes, is an essential part of everyday life for a working makeup artist. Makeup can be natural or creative, but in order for it to be good editorial makeup it must sit well within the story and not detract from it, unless it's a specific beauty story. Teamwork is essential here as there needs to be a balance for the best look.

Makeup is an art form but there are lots of technical aspects that must be deployed in order to achieve a style. You can recreate the same look over and over again, but it's the face of the model that makes the makeup look new. How the highlights and textures are placed and colour tones are used is unique to every artist. That's why you never get bored – there is always something exciting going on in the picture.

Collaborating with milliners like Louis Mariette and Justin Smith has been an amazing journey, as I am inspired by their creations. It's important to bounce ideas around to encourage outside-the-box thinking. I find it's often a new challenge when a designer comes along with a brief and you end up taking the idea elsewhere to create something different. A lot of my makeup creations and techniques come from experimenting and trying to work with someone else's brief.

Working with session hair stylists can be one of the most inspiring forms of collaboration, especially in avant-garde hairdressing, where the styles are out of this world. Makeup is used to convey a message and to enhance the overall look. If the makeup doesn't sit right it can completely ruin the hair look and potentially make the model look unattractive. There's always a balance needed and it's important that it's either statement hair or statement makeup. Having both can work, but only if they are of equal strength.

Makeup MAC Full Coverage Foundation; Face•Lace; Topshop Grunge Stick (Unkempt) Molten Eyes (Pocket Money), Chubby Liner (Bambi), Doe Eyed Lashes Mascara, Golden Aura Eye Palette **Photography** Camille Sanson **Model** Lakiza

'These images are very heartfelt and personal, a snippet of my history.'

–Louis Mariette, Milliner

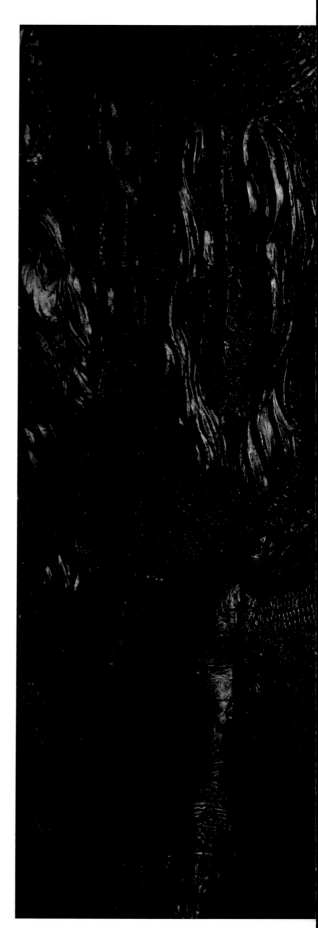

Makeup Kryolan Shimmering Event Foundation (Gold), Supracolor Interferenz (Bronze) **Photography** Camille Sanson **Headpiece** Louis Mariette **Model** Yaourou Konaté **Location** Shaka Zulu

Next page **Makeup** Kryolan Ultra Foundation Palette, Supracolor 24 Colors Palette K; brows by Iana Nohel **Photography** Camille Sanson **Hair** Diana Moar **Styling** Karl Willett **Jewellery** Vicki Sarge

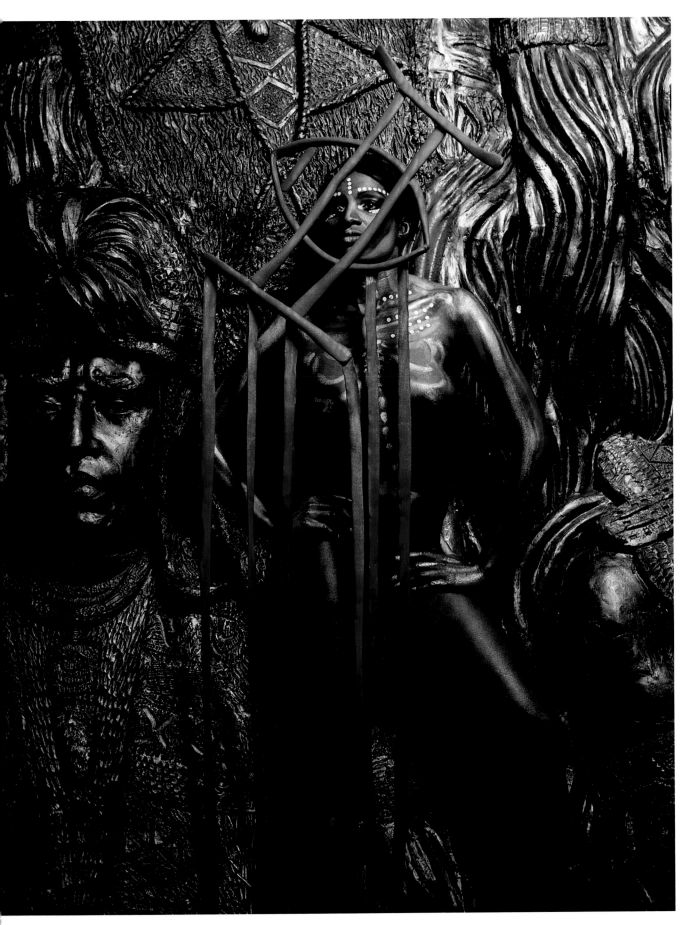

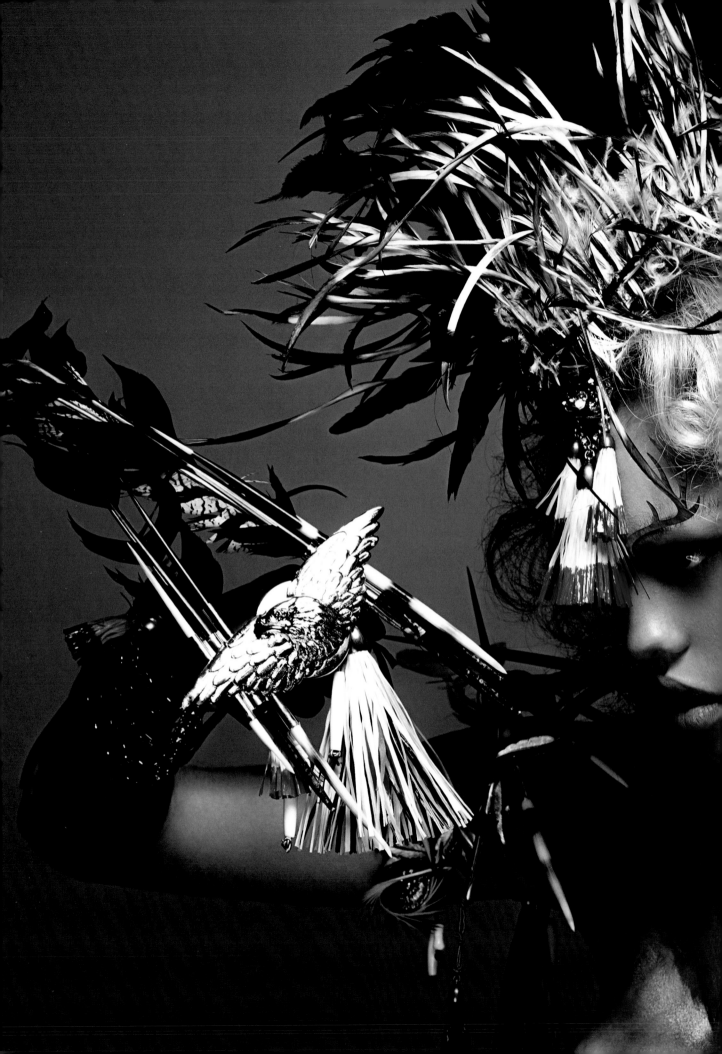

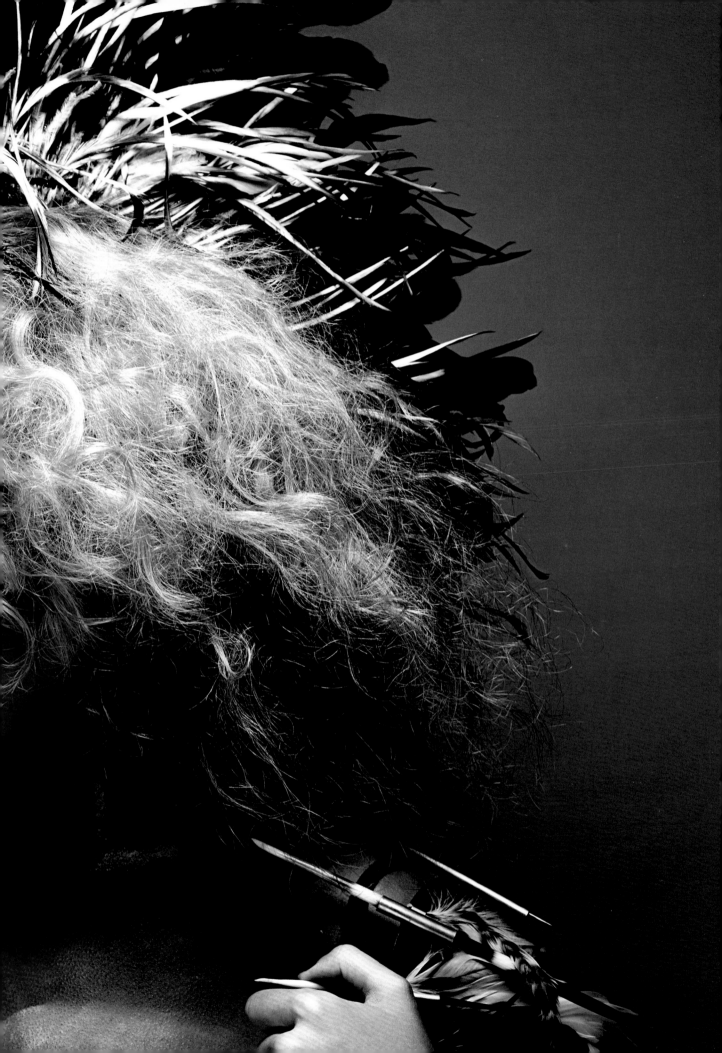

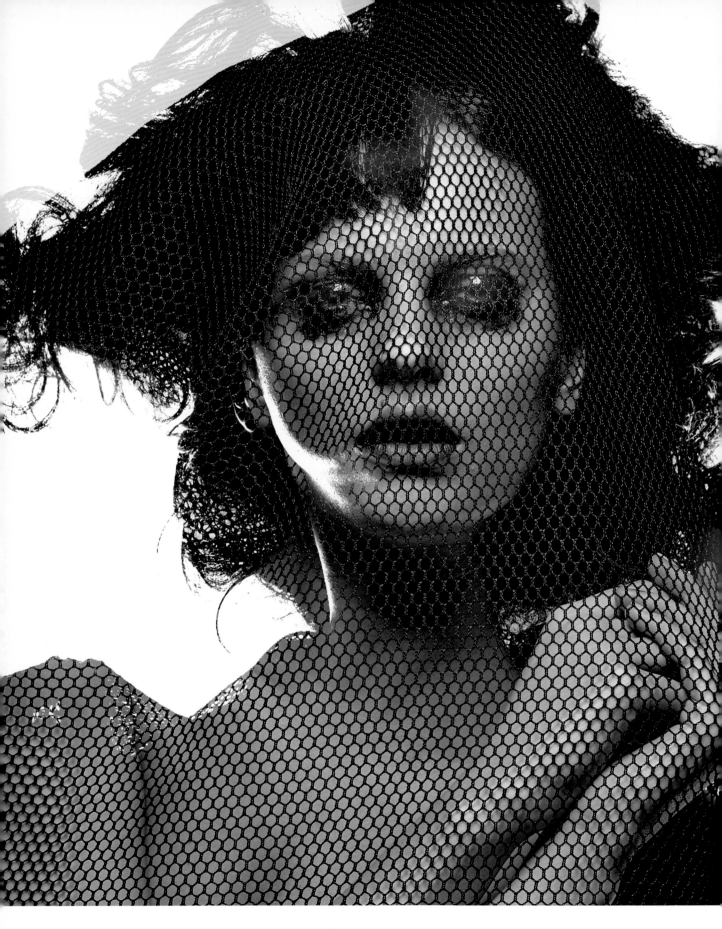

These pages **Makeup** Kryolan Supracolor
Shimmering Vision Palette, Shimmering Event
Foundation (Silver), HD Cream liner (Ebony);
Face•Lace **Photography** Camille Sanson
Hair Diana Moar using Kevin Murphy
Model (above) Barbara @ Leni's, (opposite)
Leila @ Profile

Following pages **Makeup** MAC Chromagraph
Pencil (Pure White), Eye Pencil (Ebony),
Eye Shadow (Carbon) **Photography** Camille
Sanson **Headpiece** Justin Smith **Model**
Leila @ Profile

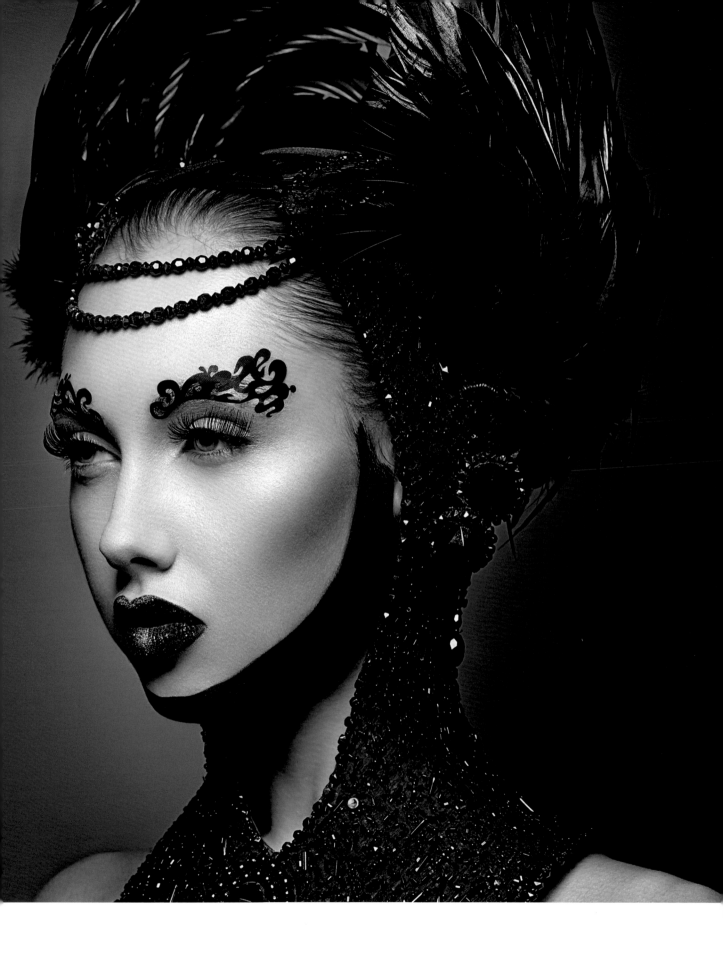

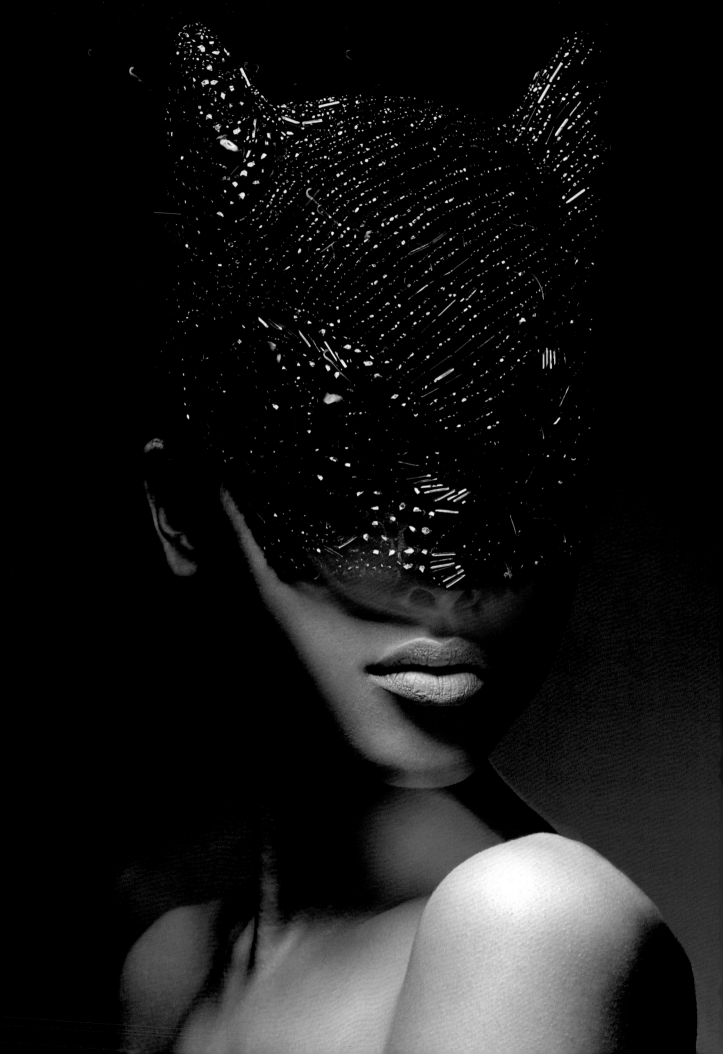

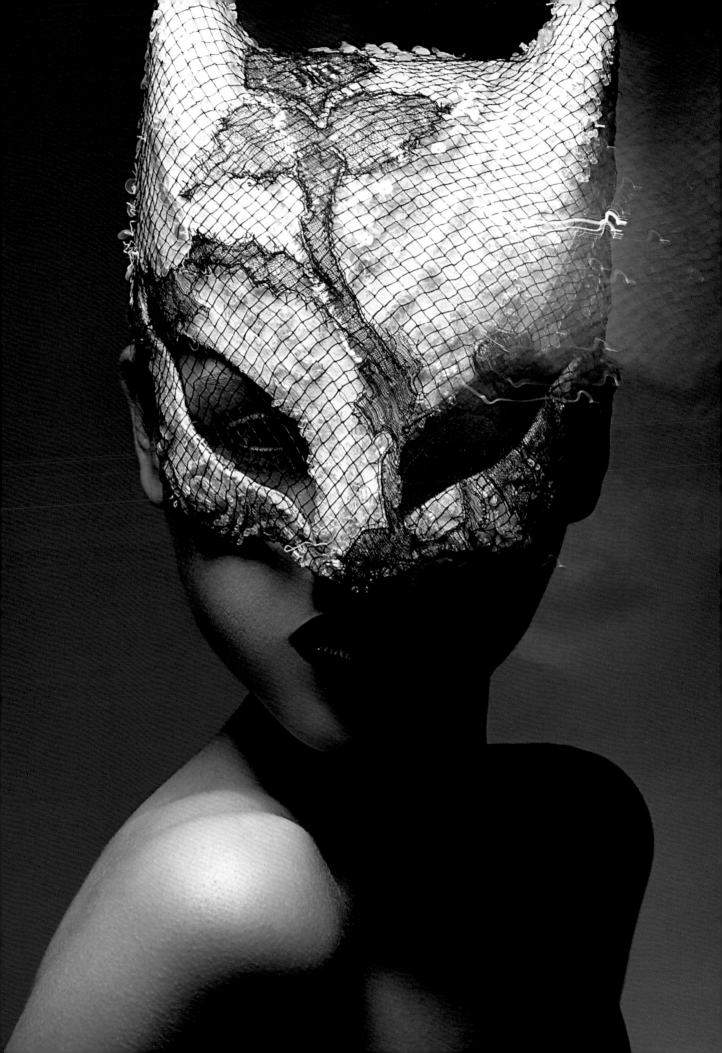

'Everything we see today has evolved throughout the decades. From the elegance and embellishments of the 1920s, and the wartorn tones and structured clothing of the 1940s and 1950s, these decades and all those in between are what allow fashion to grow and continue to push modern-day boundaries.

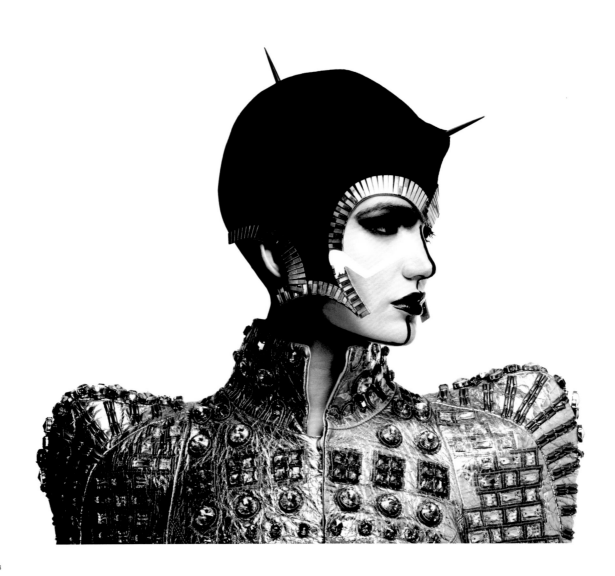

As a stylist it's important for me to understand where fashion comes from. Looking back over time, fashion has changed and moved in so many directions, but ultimately it comes back full circle, just with a fresh new approach.'

– Karl Willett, Stylist

Makeup Make Up For Ever 12 Flash Color Case, MAC Fluidline (BlackTrack); The Body Shop Colour Crush Eyeshadow (015, Moonlight Kiss) **Photography** Camille Sanson **Hair** Diana Moar **Styling** Karl Willett **Hats** Victoria Grant **Clothes** gold jacket and black dress Qasimi **Model** Mimi @ Premier **Styling Assistant** Adele Pentland

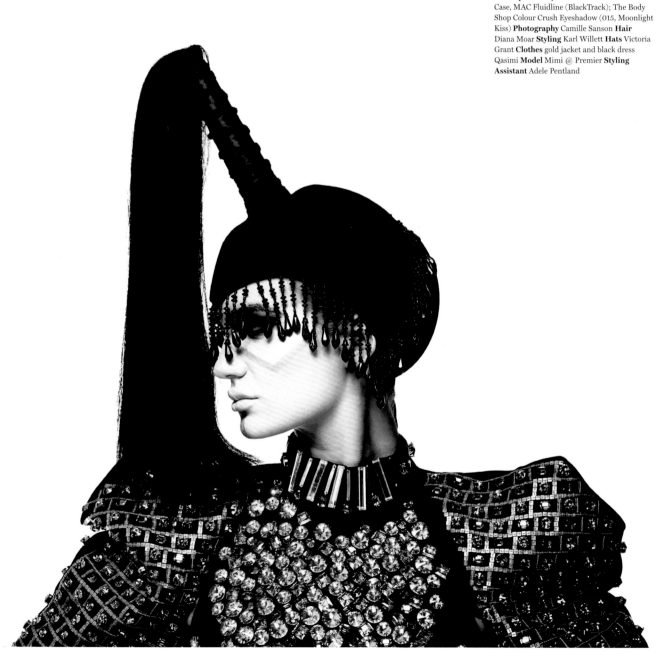

'Fashion is a painful beauty.'

– Sorapol, Fashion Designer

Makeup MAC Full Coverage Foundation;
Topshop Grunge Stick (Unkempt), Molten Eyes
(Pocket Money), Chubby Liner (Bambi), Doe
Eyed Lashes Mascara, Golden Aura Eye
Palette; Face•Lace **Photography** Camille
Sanson **Hair** Diana Moar **Styling** Karl Willett
Clothes Sorapol **Model** Lakiza **Styling**
Assistant Adele Pentland **Nails** The Freelance
Workspace using Essie

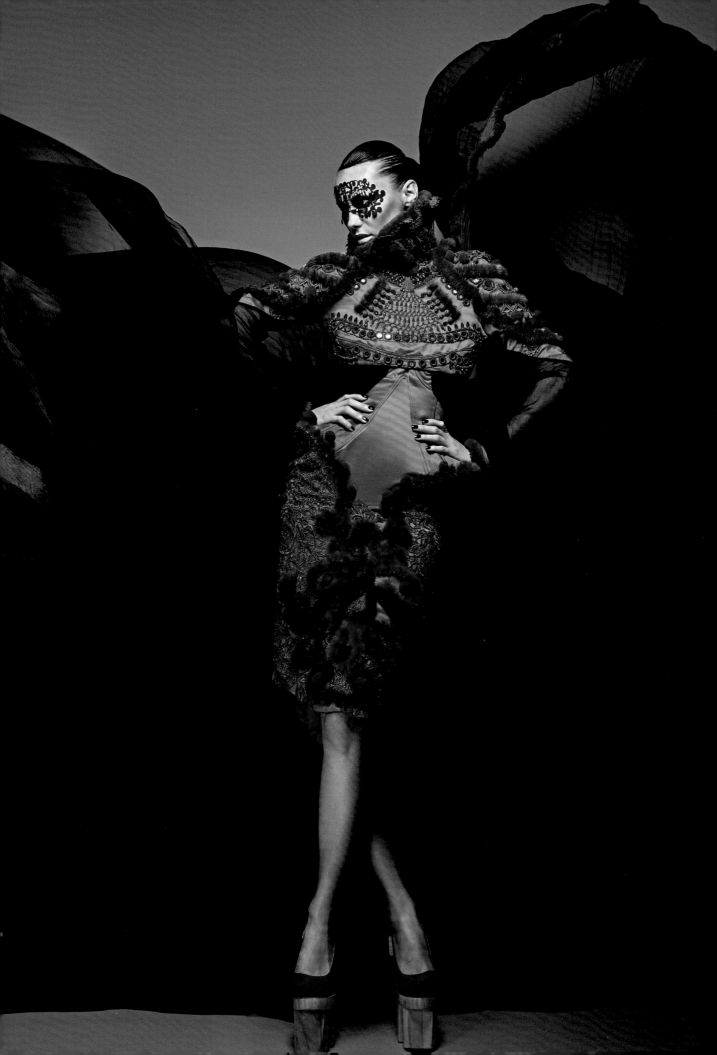

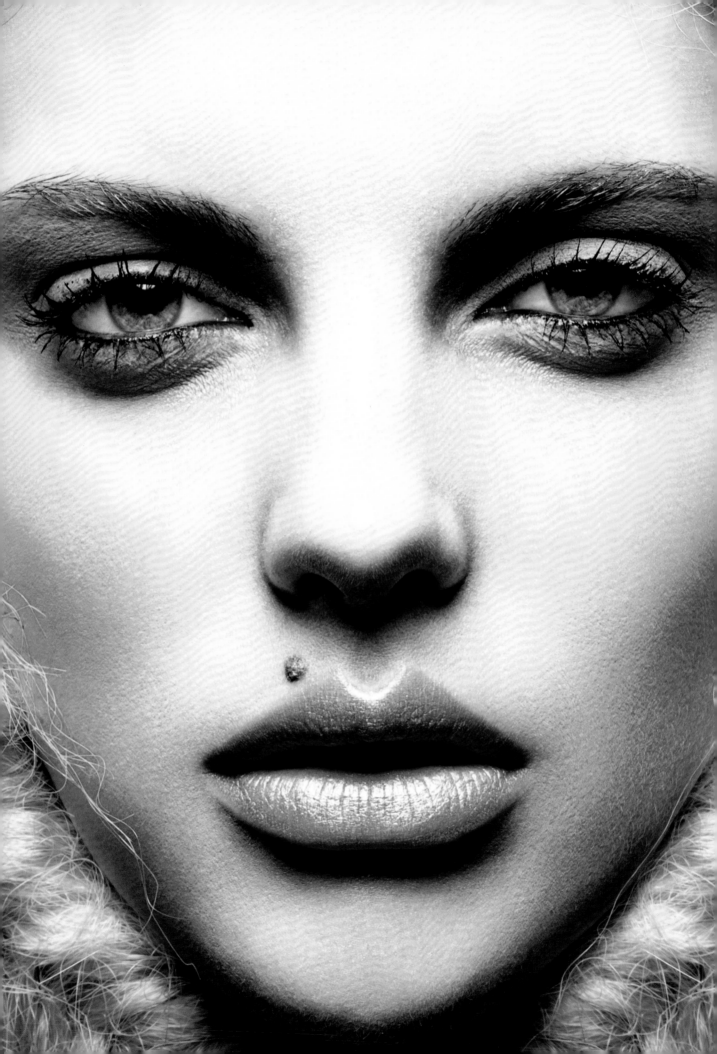

6. My Magic Formula

Texture, lips, eyes, get the look

'I believe that it is the chemists who make the products that are the innovators. They allow me to create new looks and reinvent old ones because of the new textures and colours.'

Texture

Textures affect the finish of the overall look, for example the skin being dewy, glossy, matt, velvet or mineral. Today's formulations contain ingredients and technologies that have been scientifically proven to nourish and protect the skin. Texture is important as it helps to define the look and create an ambience, whether applied on skin, eyes or lips. Different textures help to highlight and draw attention to certain areas of the face.

Layering up textures is an important skill when developing a look as it adds extra dimensions. Using wet-to-dry products has been a big development in makeup art and there is a lot of choice when it comes to cream bases, powders and, more recently, velvety finishes in the products.

Mineral makeup is a loose powder form that is made from natural pigments. It is light in texture, and is generally brushed on to the skin.

Previous page **Makeup** The Body Shop All-In-One BB Cream, Moisture Foundation, Lightening Touch, Colour Crush Eyeshadows (001, Sugar Glaze; 240, Gorgeous Gold; 301, Pink Crush; 310, Berry Cheeky; 401, Lavender Love; 410, Blackcurrant Affair), Divide and Multiply Mascara, Eye Definer (01, Black), Shimmer Cube Palette (Purple), All-In-One Cheek Colour (Macaroon), Colour Crush Lipstick (245, Pink Luxe) **Photography** Camille Sanson **Hair** Diana Moar using Bumble and Bumble **Model** Barbara @ Leni's

Opposite **Makeup** Givenchy Magic Kajal Eye Pencil; MAC Eye Shadow (Idol Eyes); Tom Ford Lip Color (Nude Vanille); Clarins Beauty Flash Balm; Yves Saint Laurent Le Teint Touche Éclat Foundation **Photography** Camille Sanson **Hair** Diana Moar **Post-production** Katrin Straupe **Nails** Pebbles Aikens using Tom Ford Nail Lacquer (Coral Blame)

Following pages (left) **Makeup** MAC Black Track Cake liner, Pigments (Ruby Red, Marine Ultra) Glitters (Reflects Red, Reflects Turquatic); Sisley Phyto-Lip Star **Photography** Camille Sanson

(right) **Makeup** MAC Lipstick (Russian Red), Lip Pencil (Redd); Giorgio Armani Lip Maestro (700 Color Zero) **Photography** Camille Sanson **Nails** Pebbles Aikens using Tom Ford Nail Lacquer (Bordeaux Lust, Carnal Red)

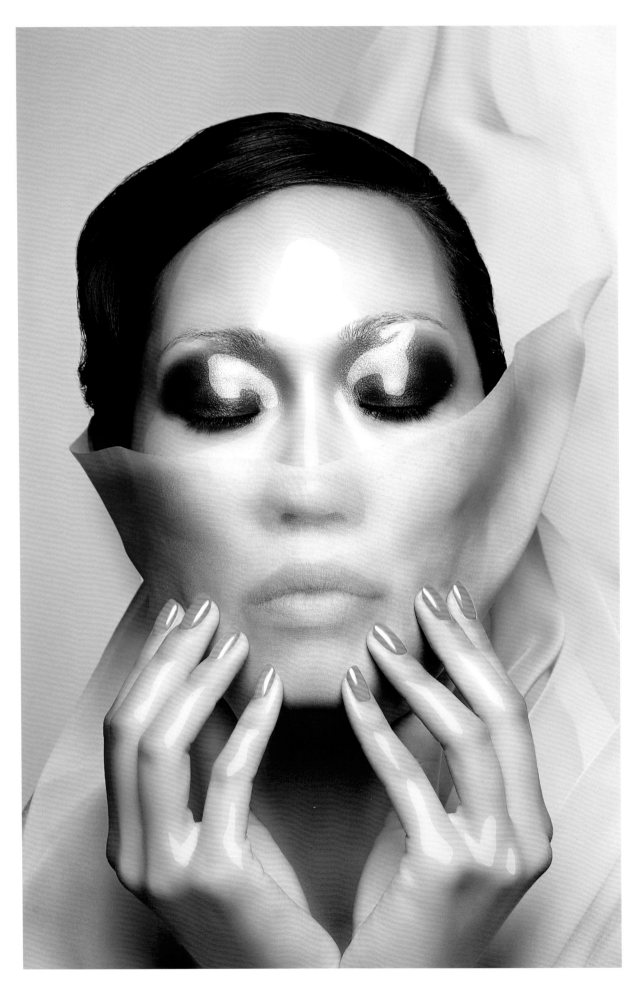

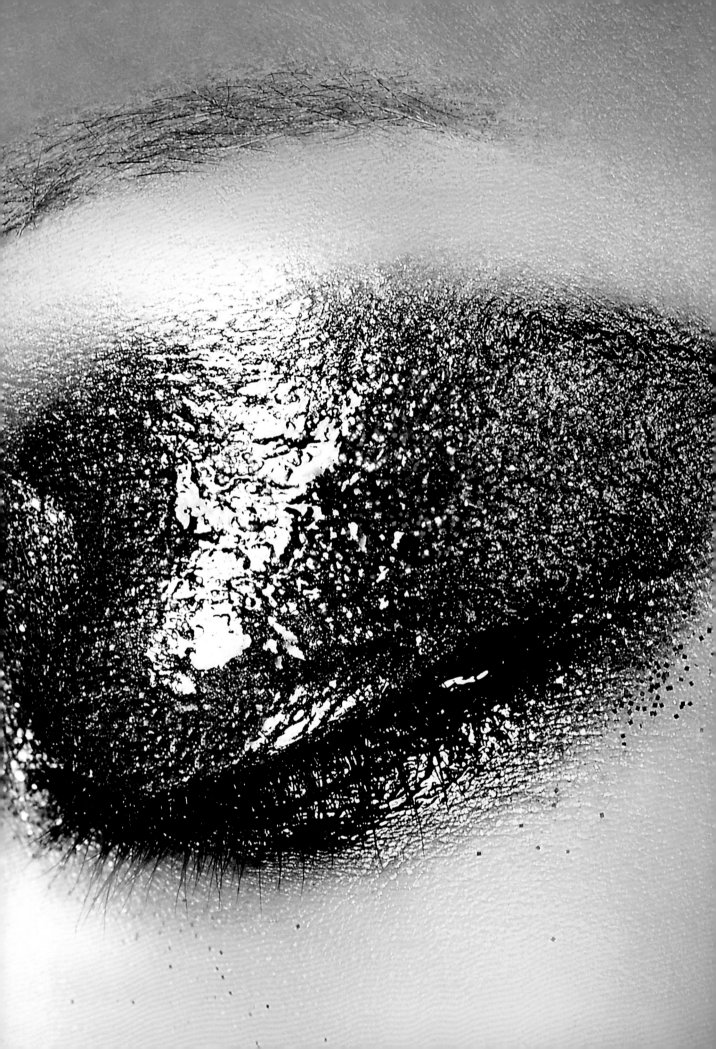

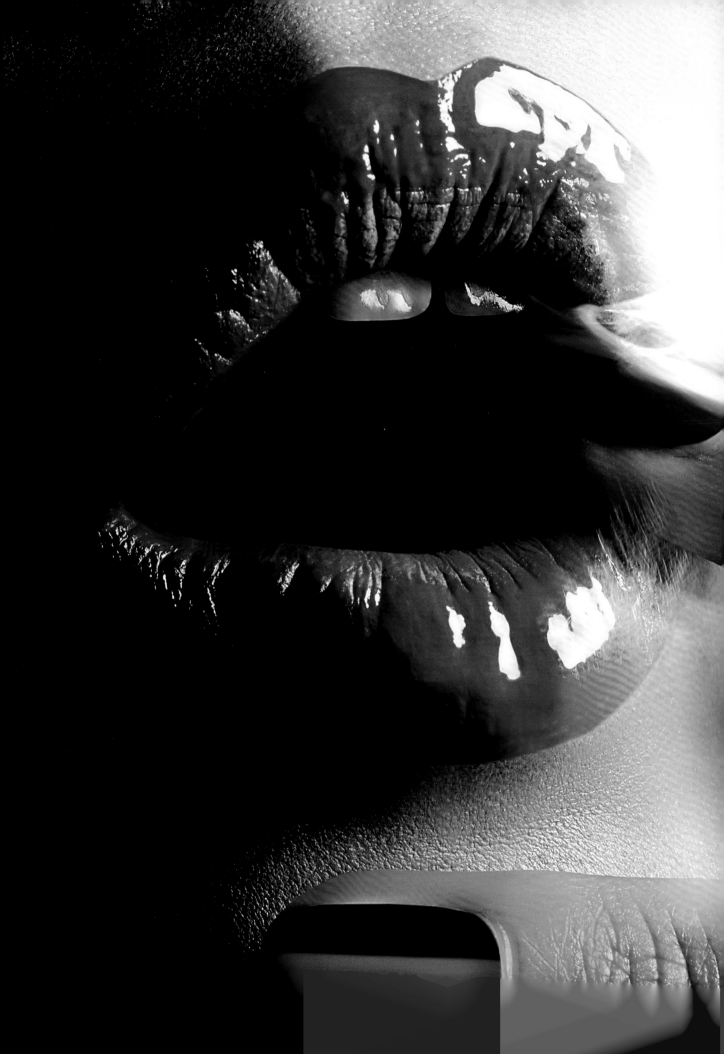

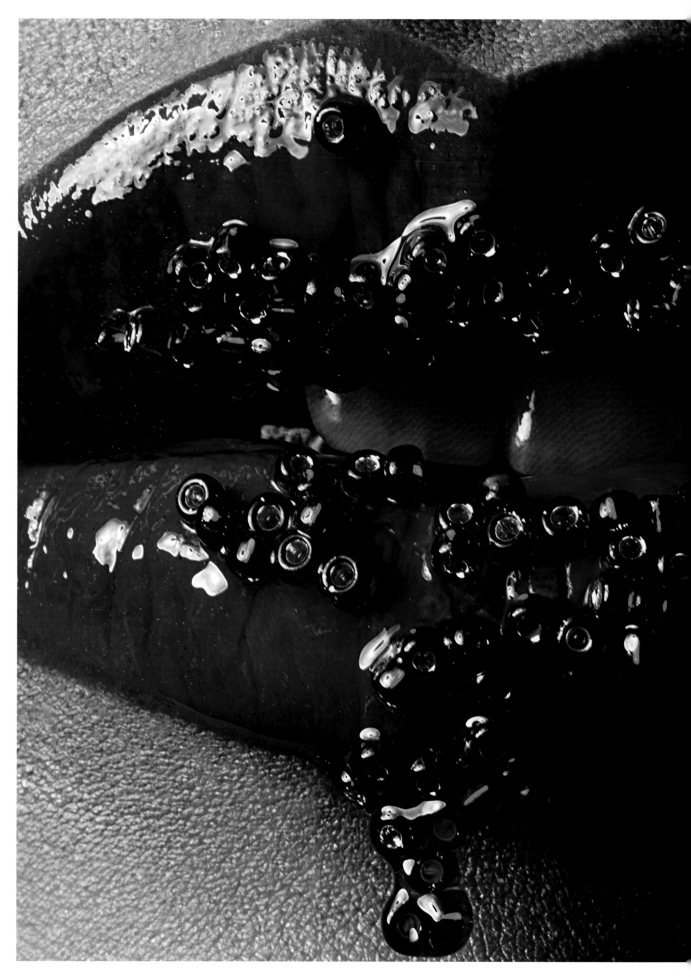

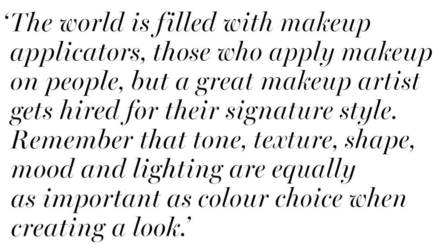

'The world is filled with makeup applicators, those who apply makeup on people, but a great makeup artist gets hired for their signature style. Remember that tone, texture, shape, mood and lighting are equally as important as colour choice when creating a look.'

– Rachel Wood, Celebrity Makeup Artist & Beauty Journalist
www.mascaramemories.com

Makeup Rouge Dior (999), Dior Addict Fluid
Stick (754, Pandore); **Photography** Catherine
Harbour

'*Beautiful Movements Cosmetics is a cruelty-free, natural, mineral-based makeup choice that offers beautiful pops of colour and flawless coverage. The line helps support a perfect complexion with zinc oxide, aloe vera and jojoba oil.*'

– Kimberly Wyatt, CEO,
  Beautiful Movements Cosmetics

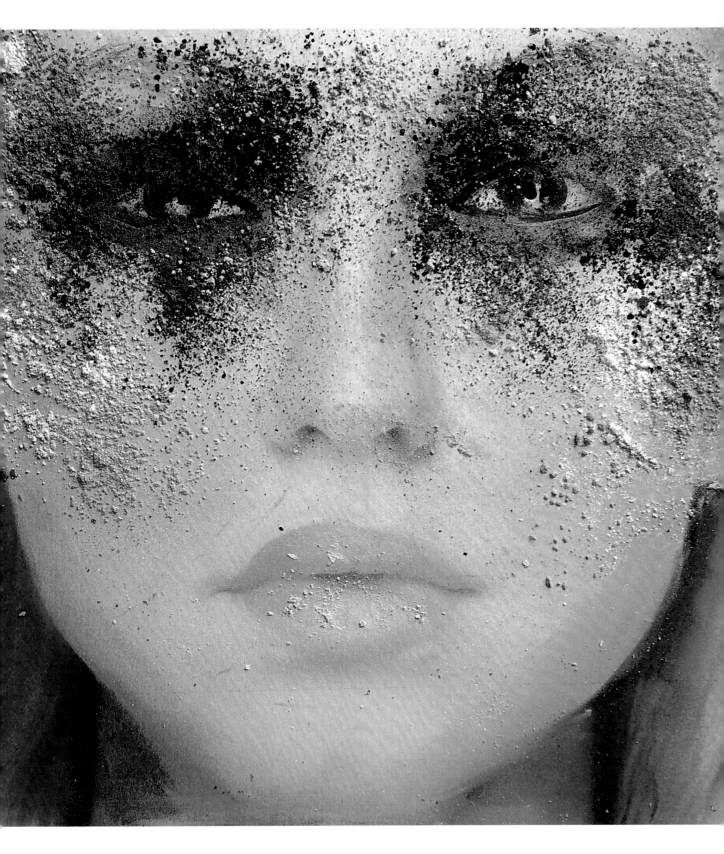

Above Lan's smudge chart using Beautiful
Movements Cosmetics

Following page **Makeup** Kryolan HD
Cream Liner (Ebony), Kajal Pencil (Black),
UV-Dayglow Compact Color Palette
Photography Catherine Harbour

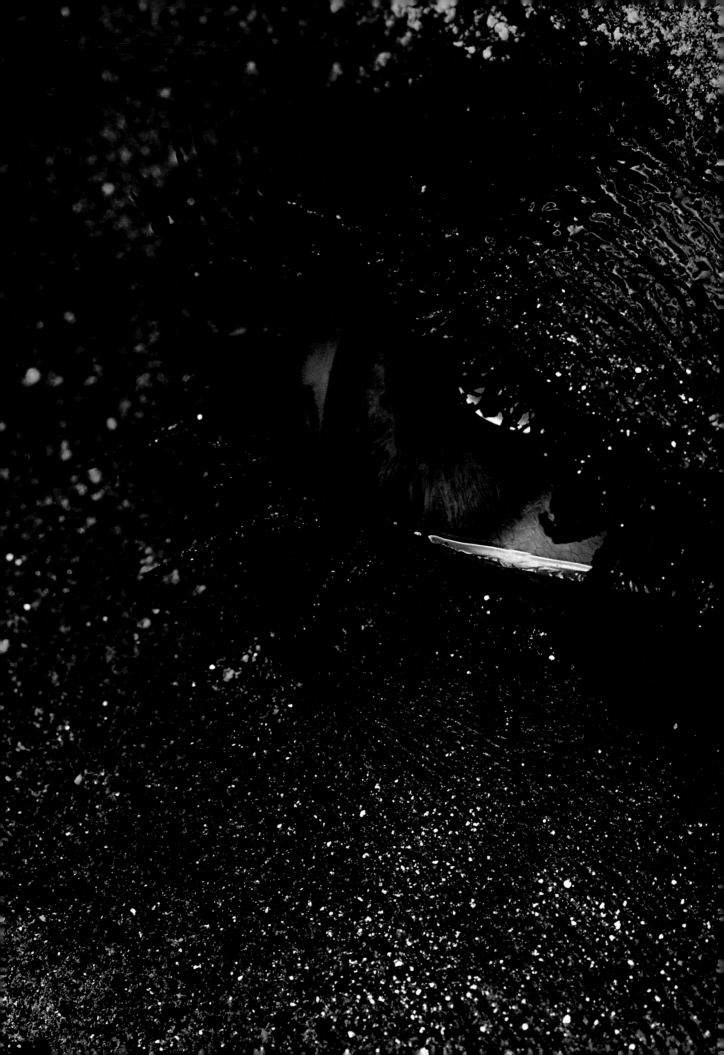

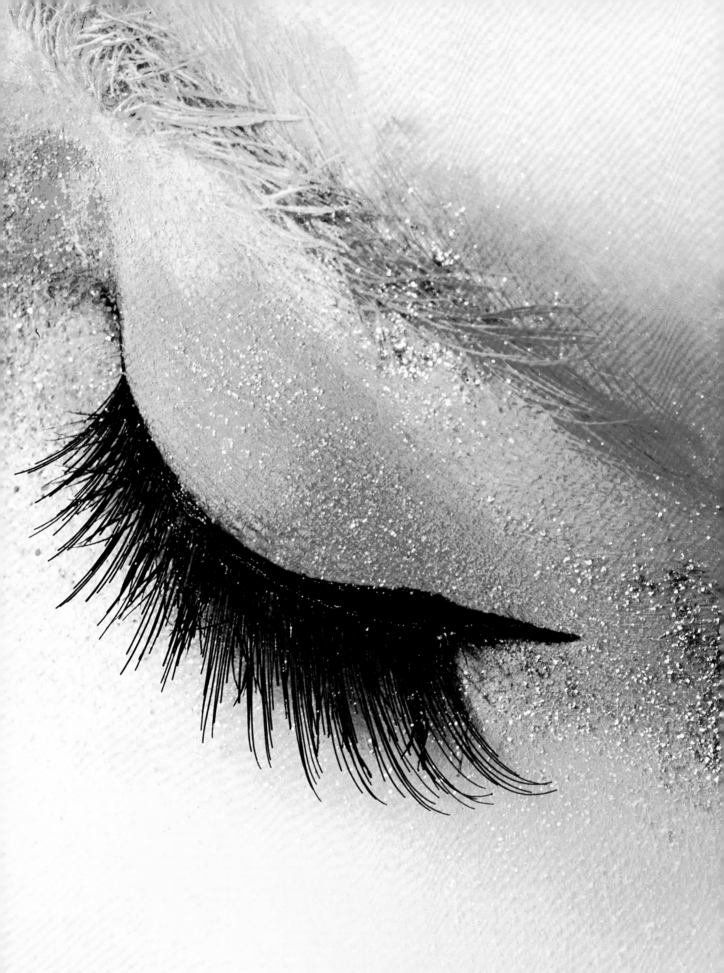

Makeup Kryolan UV-Dayglow Compact Color
Palette, HD Cream Liner (Ebony)
Photography Mark Cant **Model** Ellie

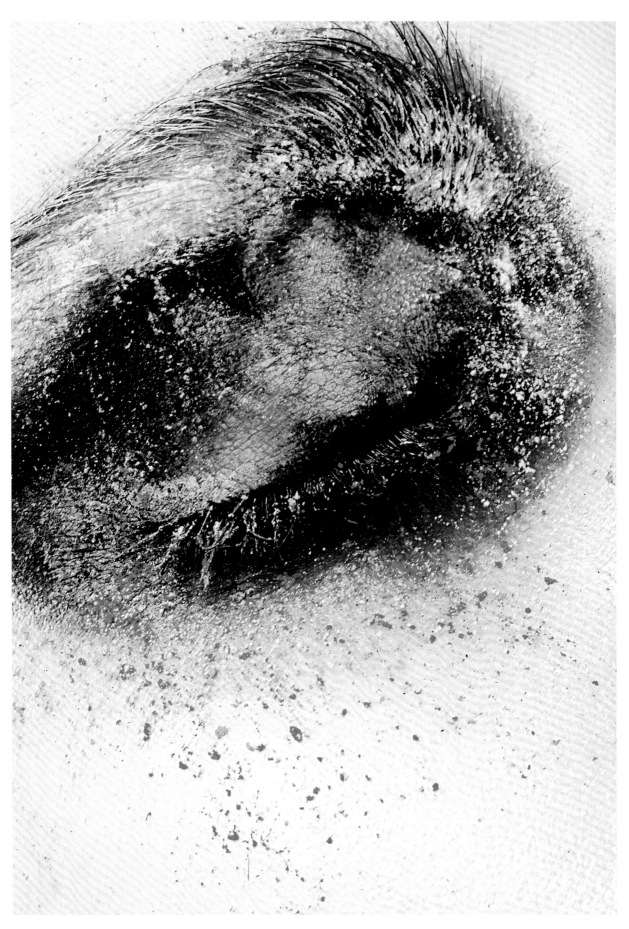

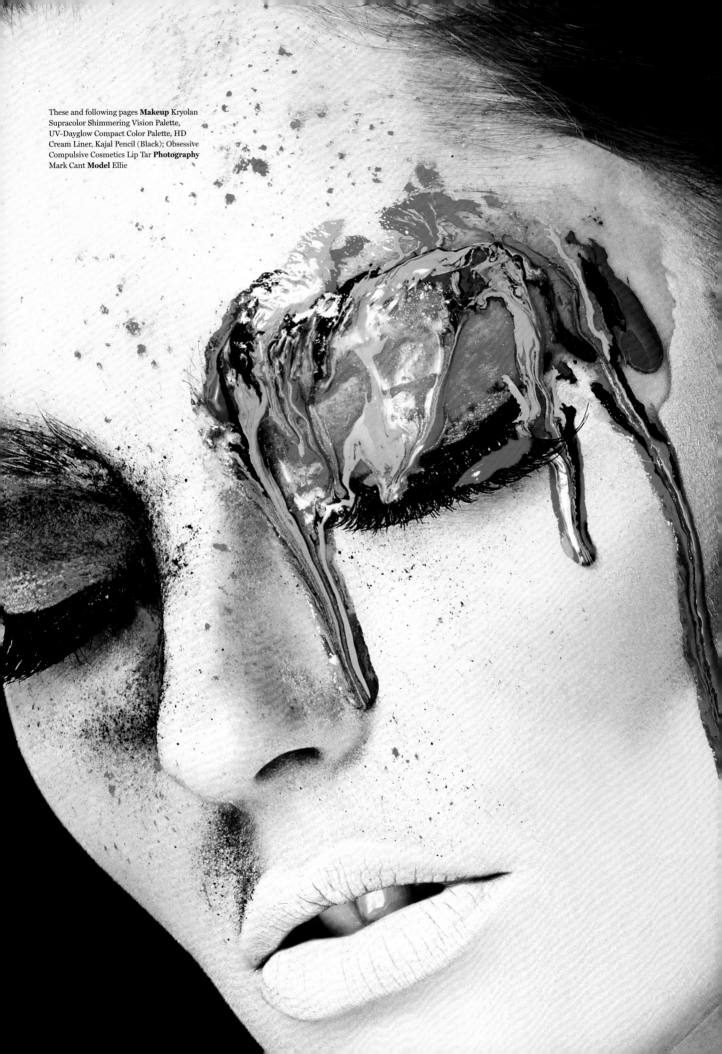

These and following pages **Makeup** Kryolan
Supracolor Shimmering Vision Palette,
UV-Dayglow Compact Color Palette, HD
Cream Liner, Kajal Pencil (Black); Obsessive
Compulsive Cosmetics Lip Tar **Photography**
Mark Cant **Model** Ellie

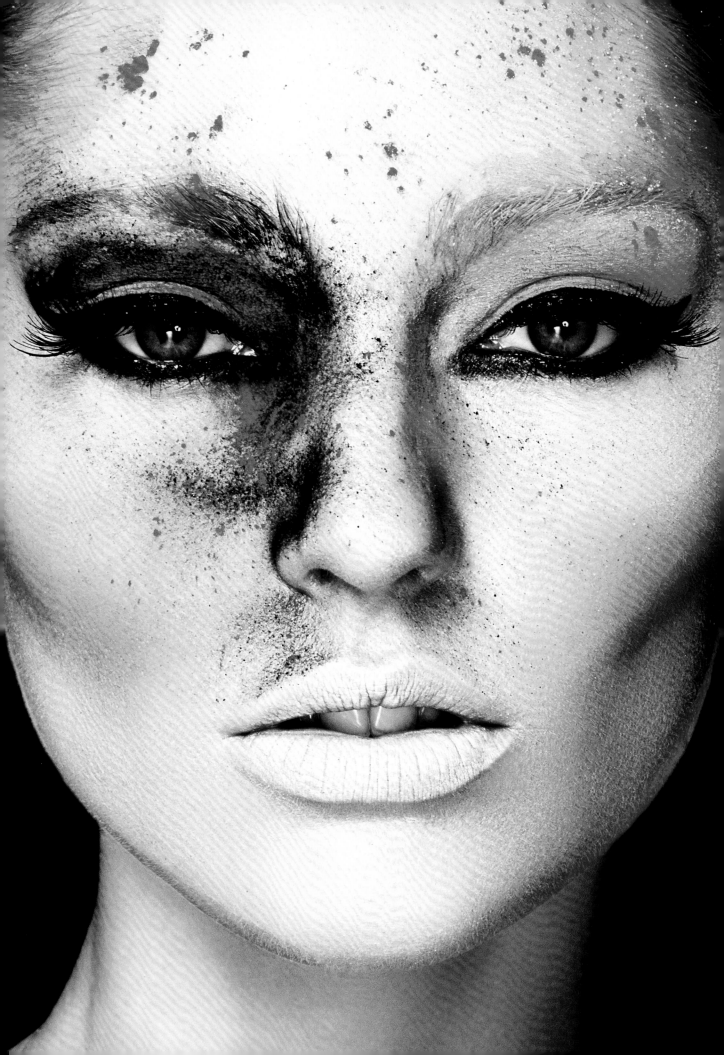

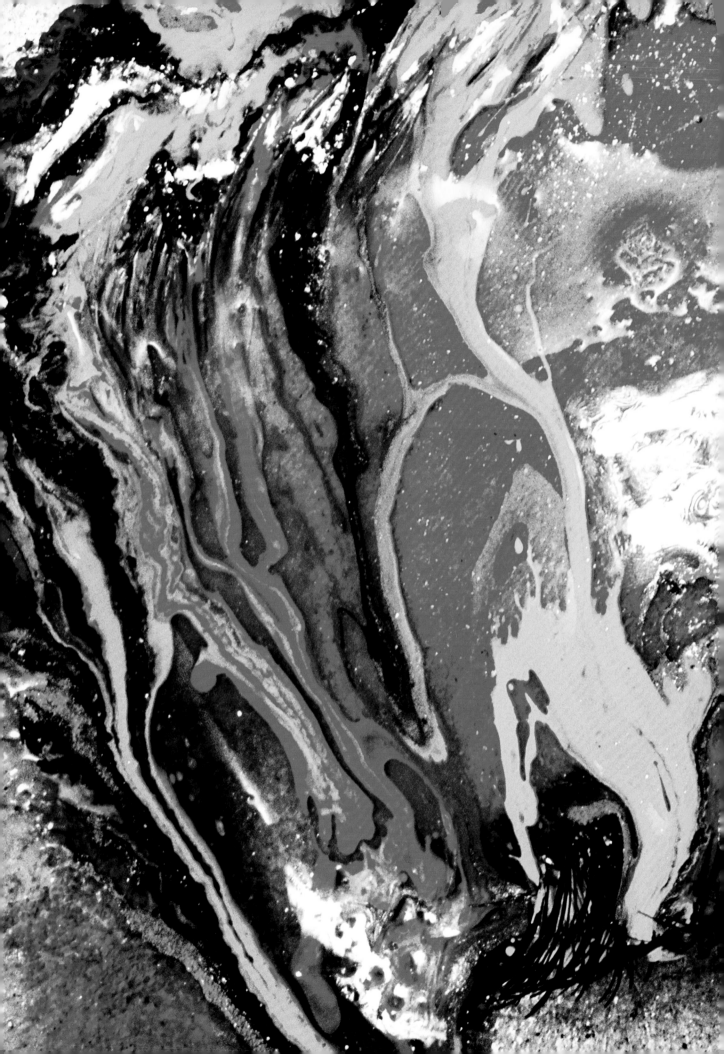

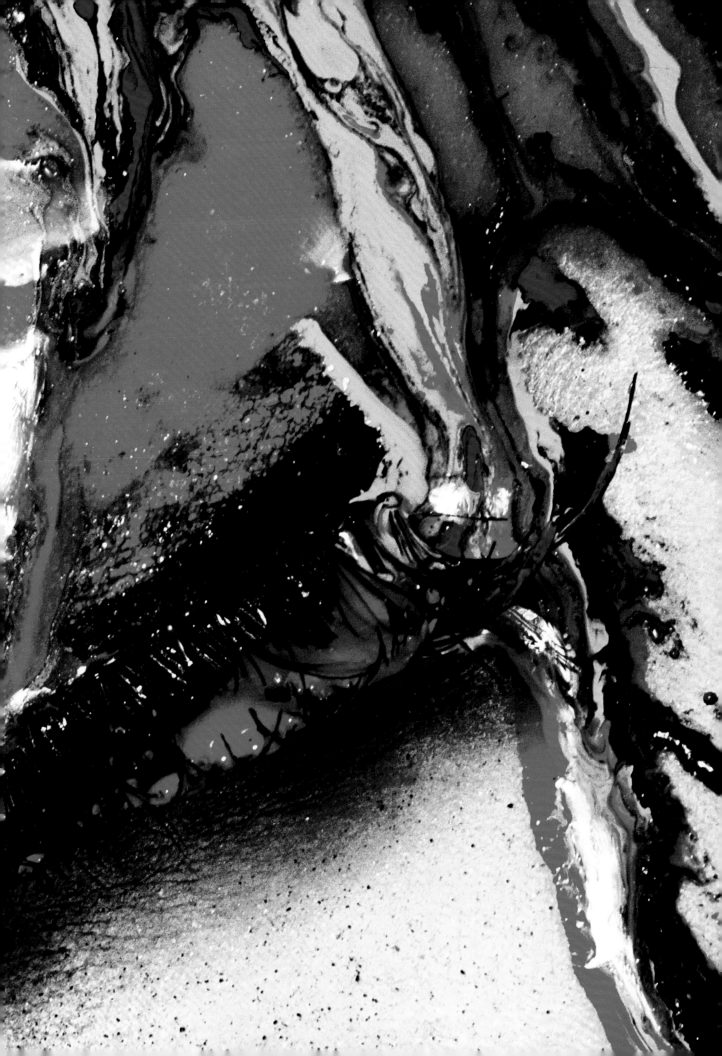

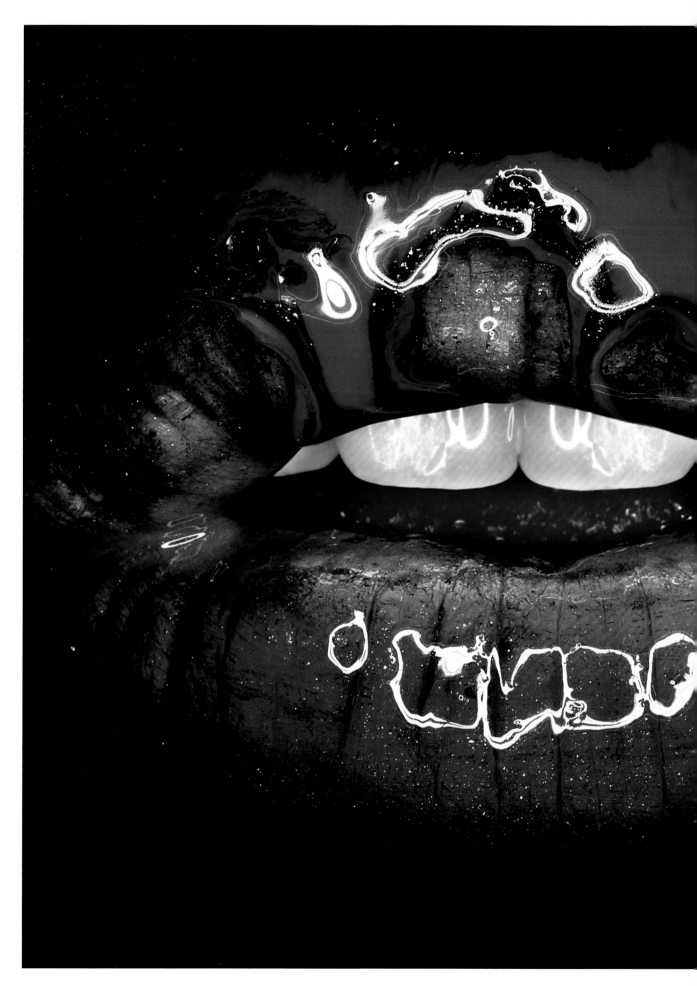

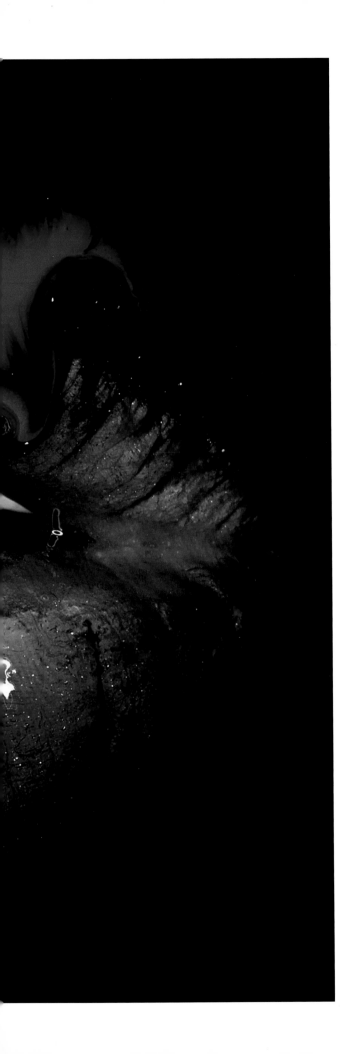

Lips

Lip shades and textures have the capacity to anchor an entire look. Synonymous with Hollywood glamour, the classic red lip had its iconic status cemented by the film industry elite of the 1940s and, like the little black dress, has recurred across history to achieve genuine timelessness. Paired with a feline flick of liner, wide-eyed Marilyn-esque lashes and a well-groomed brow, the boldly rouged, highly pigmented lip achieves immediate visual impact.

Begin with a lip liner slightly darker than your choice of lipstick, working outwards from your cupid's bow to define the shape of your mouth. Shading the whole lip with the lip liner provides a long-lasting base. Hues that offer a contemporary edge include pigmented neon reds and two-toned orange–red hybrids. A shimmer pigment is best if you want to shape and contour thinner lips, while a matt finish works better on a naturally full mouth. Don't be afraid to mix your own unique shade of red – there is a red lip to suit everyone; just make sure you match the base with your skin tone. As a general rule, lipsticks with yellow and orange undertones suit warmer skin tones, while cooler complexions respond well to blue-toned reds. Be brave in your application; a modestly applied, indefinite colour can end up washing you out.

For a sense of luxuriousness, there are two possible avenues: a chic, matt finish or a glossy, vampiric lip. Applying a finishing touch of powder to lipstick attains a demure, semi-matt aesthetic that works well for daytime and office wear. A layer of gloss, conversely, will completely change the feel of the lip, amping up the volume for a fuller feel. Sometimes just adding a dot to the centre of the cupid's bow is enough to give that super-doll shape. Choose a clear gloss if you want to play safe, or a highly pigmented coloured gloss if you want to experiment.

Makeup Make Up For Ever 12 Flash Color Case; MAC Lipglass; Obsessive Compulsive Cosmetics Lip Tar **Photography** John Oakley

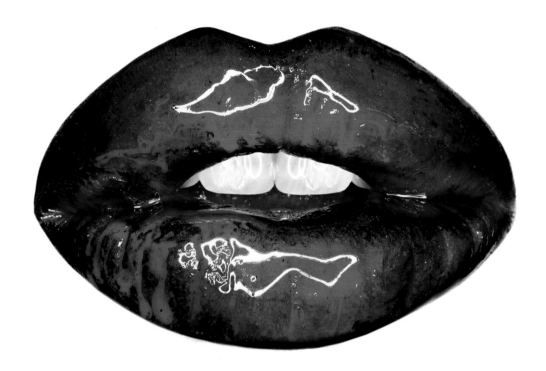

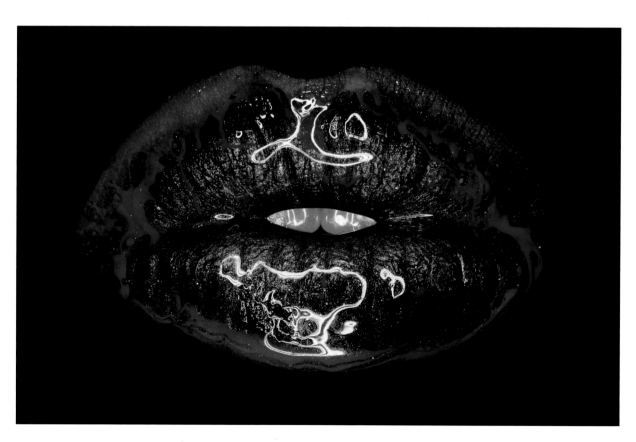

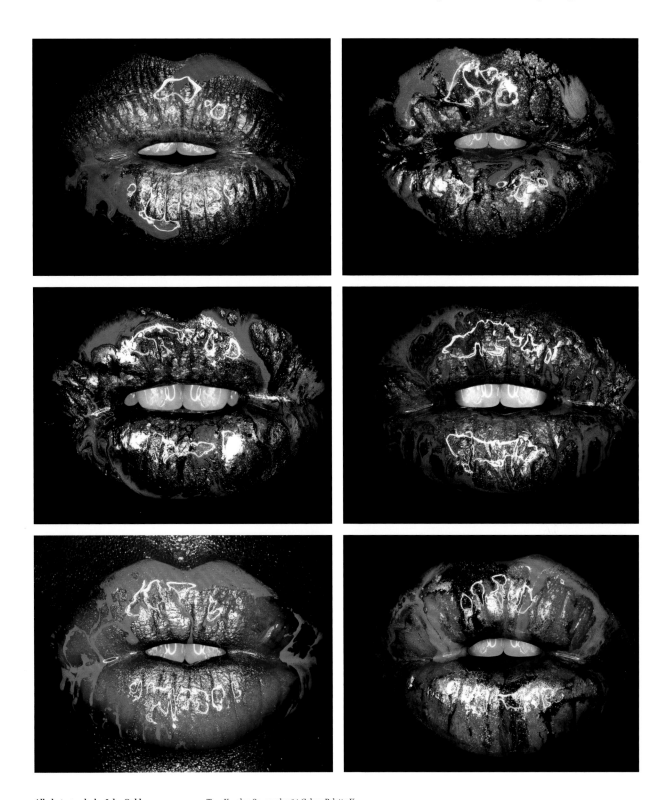

All photography by John Oakley

Opposite: Giorgio Armani Lip Maestro (401, Tibetan Orange), Flash Lacquer (102)

Top: Kryolan Supracolor 24 Colors Palette K, Glamour Sparks, UV Color Paints, Liquid Color Paints, Multi Gel Glitter, Supracolor Shimmering Vision Palette, Aquacolor Glitter Paint

Middle: MAC Fluidline (Blacktrack), Glitters (Reflects Purple Duo, Reflects Pearl, Reflects Turquatic, Amethyst), Lipglass

Bottom: (left) Bourjois Rouge Edition Velvet (03, Hot Pepper), Aqua Rouge Edition Aqua Shades, Red My Lips, Intense Eyeshadow (10) (right) Bourjois Rouge Edition Velvet (06, Ping Pong), Aqua in Fuchsia Perche

'*The beauty industry relies on a desire to enhance reality. As digital technology advances, the gap between fantasy and reality expands. New expectations of more spectacular versions of ourselves will create the need for minimum effort with maximum result products.*'

– Phyllis Cohen, Makeup Artist

Below **Makeup** MAC Powerpoint Eye Pencils (So There Jade, Prussian), Glitters (Reflects Purple Duo, Reflects Turquatic, 3D Brass Gold, 3D Lavender, 3D Pink, 3D Silver) **Photography** Mark Cant

Opposite **Makeup** Kryolan Supracolor Shimmering Vision Palette, Multi Gel Glitter, Eye Shadow Glitter **Photography** Mark Cant **Model** Ellie

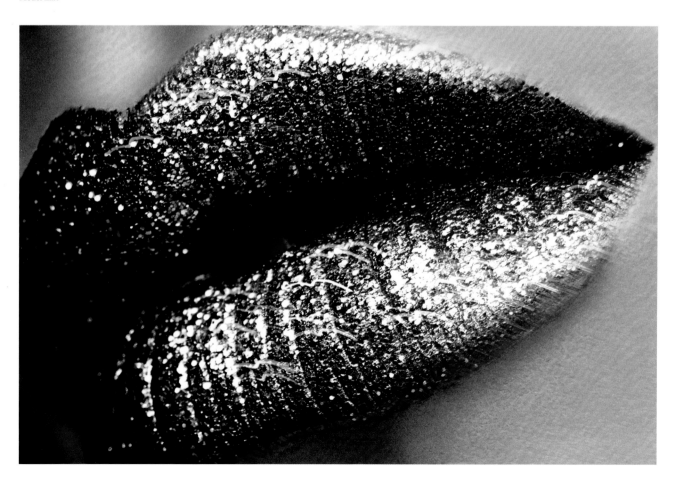

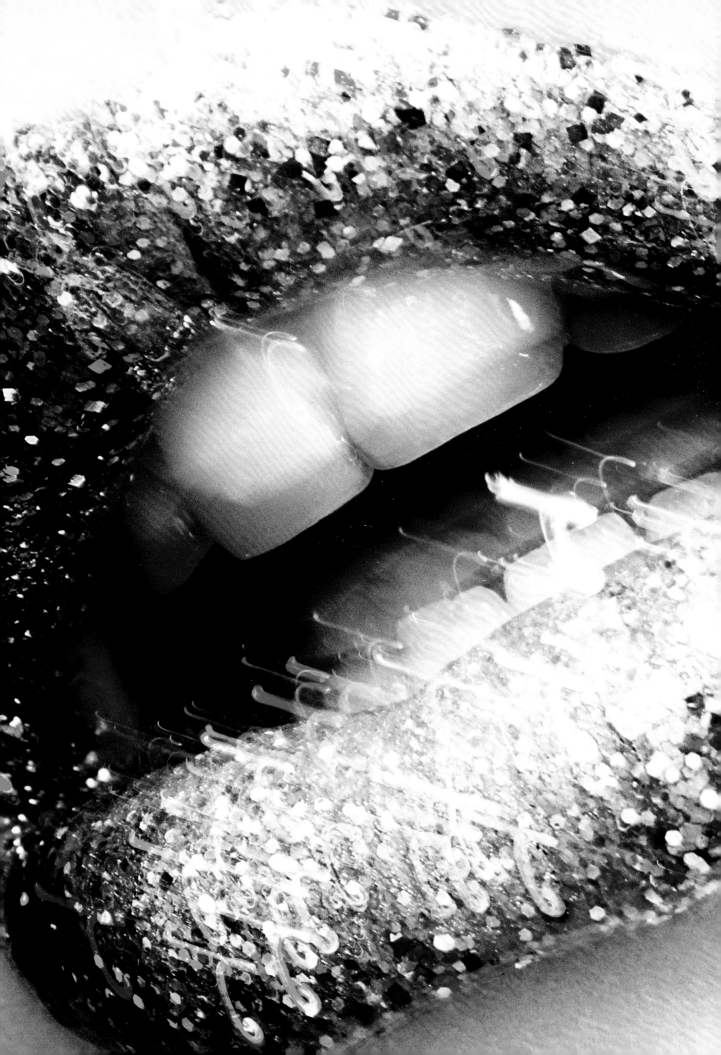

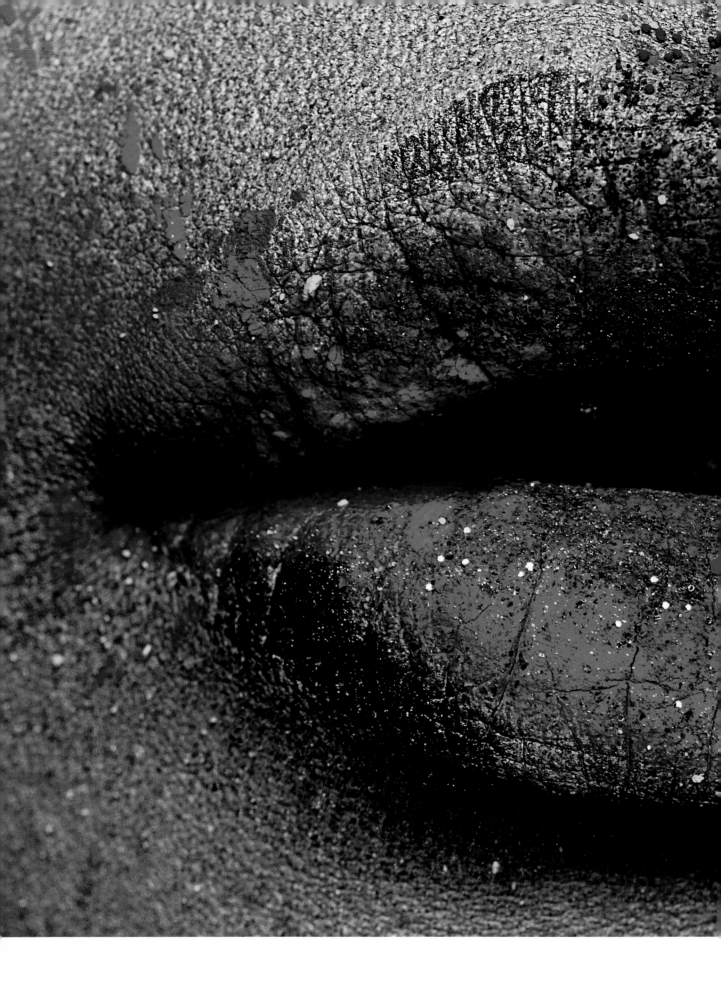

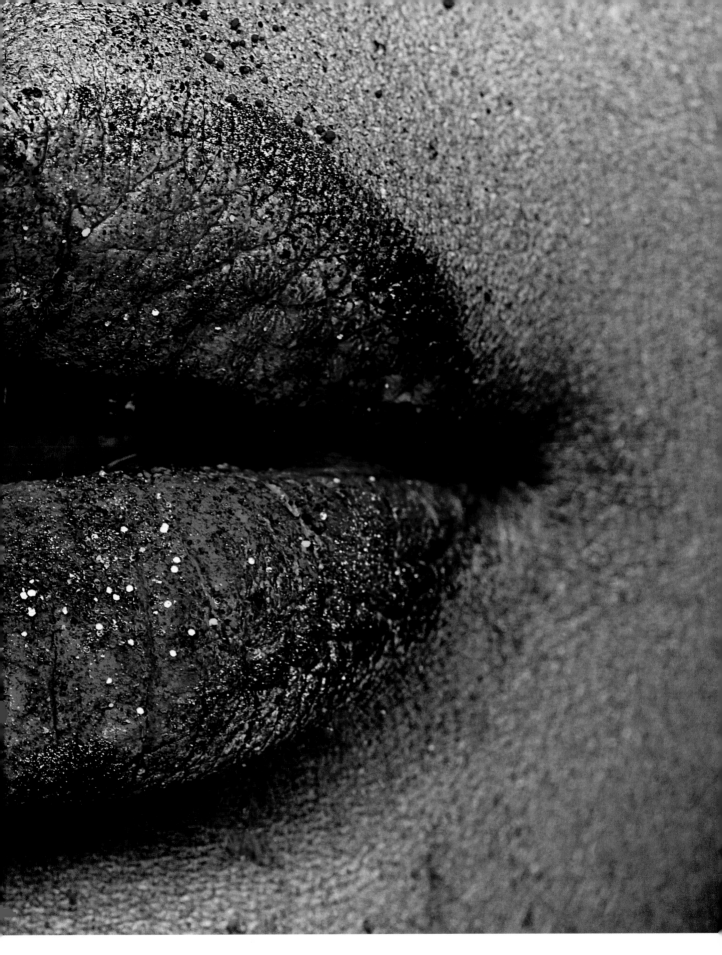

Above **Makeup** Kryolan UV-Dayglow Compact
Color Palette **Photography** Catherine Harbour

Following page **Makeup** Kryolan UV-Dayglow
Compact Color Palette **Photography** John Oakley

177

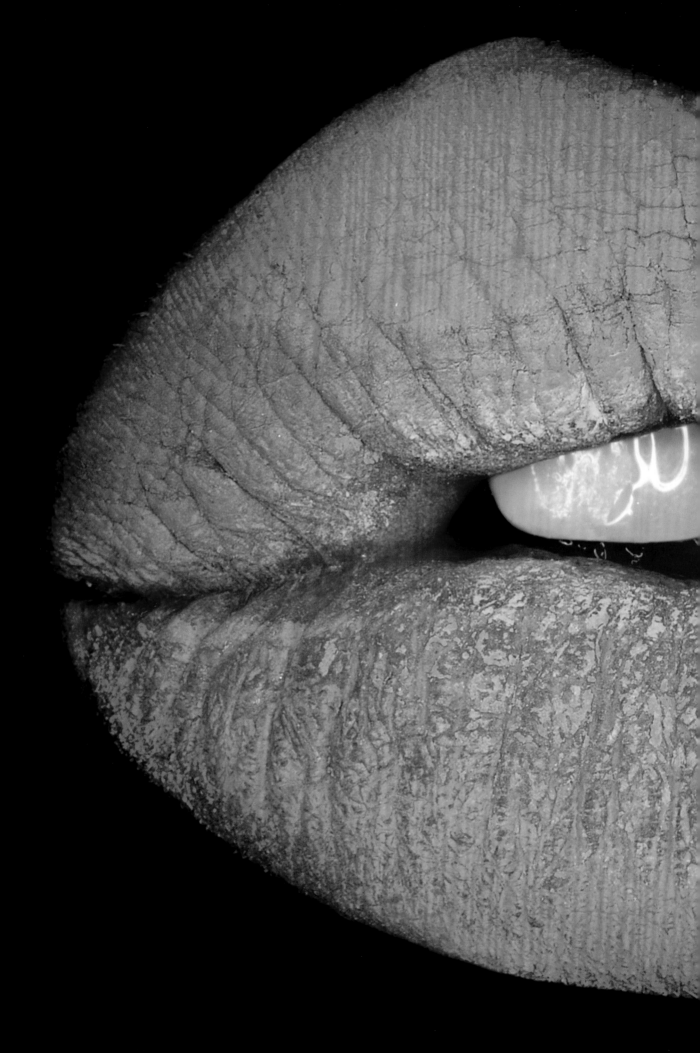

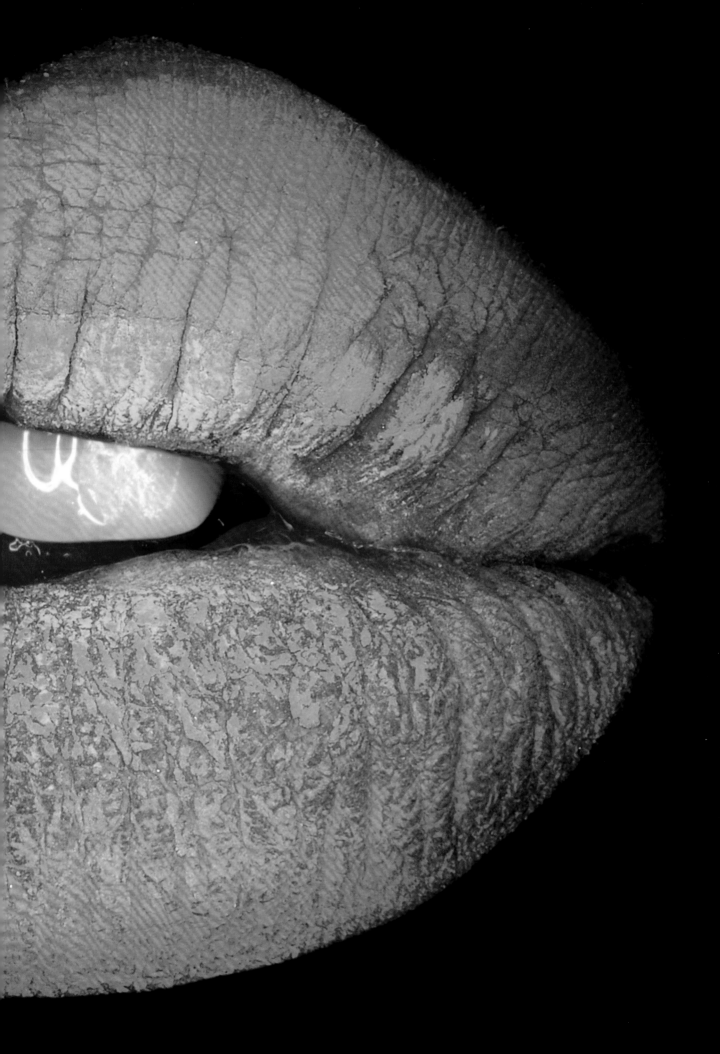

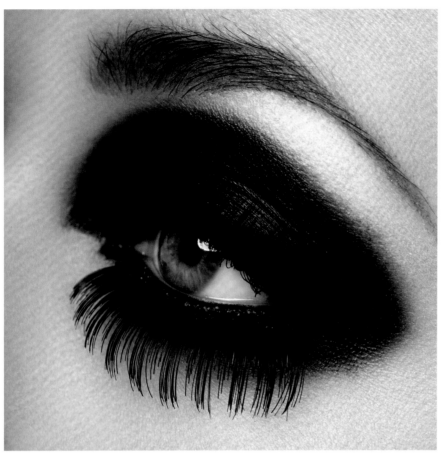

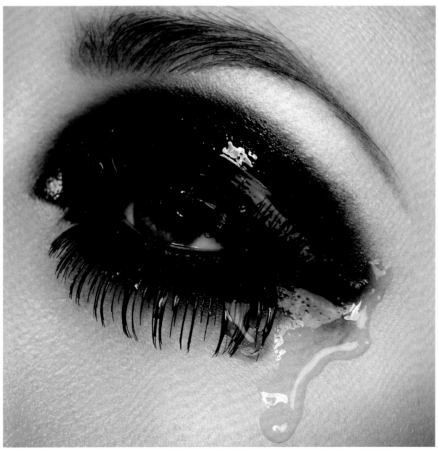

Defining the eyes

It may sound obvious, but if you want to create graphic black eye makeup, be certain that the eyeshadow you choose is actually black – there are lots of beauty-counter options specified as 'black' that have blue and grey tones, which when applied look too light. Often I apply a layer of cream black gel with a greasepaint consistency, before setting with black powder on top. As well as lasting longer, this is a failsafe route to achieving depth of colour.

Perfecting the perfect swoop of eyeliner takes time and practise. Start by mapping out the line with a kohl pencil or thin, flat eyeshadow brush, then build up the line little by little until you're confident enough to do a straight sweep over the top. Choose a gel or waterproof liquid formula for a longer-lasting finish. If you have oilier skin, you can always set your liner with a little powder to prevent it from smudging. When creating a 1960s smoky eye à la Twiggy, powder is essential, as the clean line within the socket can fade easily.

Of course, your eyeliner needn't always be precise – softly smudging dark kohl liner towards the outer corners of your eyes results in a sexy, dishevelled grunge look. In terms of your eye shape, a touch of white liner will widen almond-shaped eyes, while winged shapes give a cat-like prowess and lift droopy eyes.

Makeup MAC Fluidline (Blacktrack), Eye Kohl (Smolder), Haute & Naughty Lash Mascara, 6 Lash eyelashes, 12 Lash eyelashes, Gloss Crème Brilliance **Photography** Mark Cant

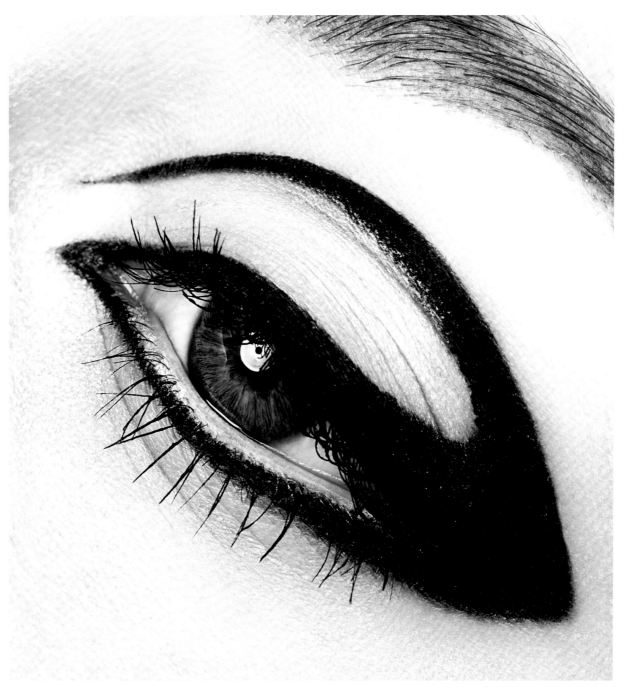

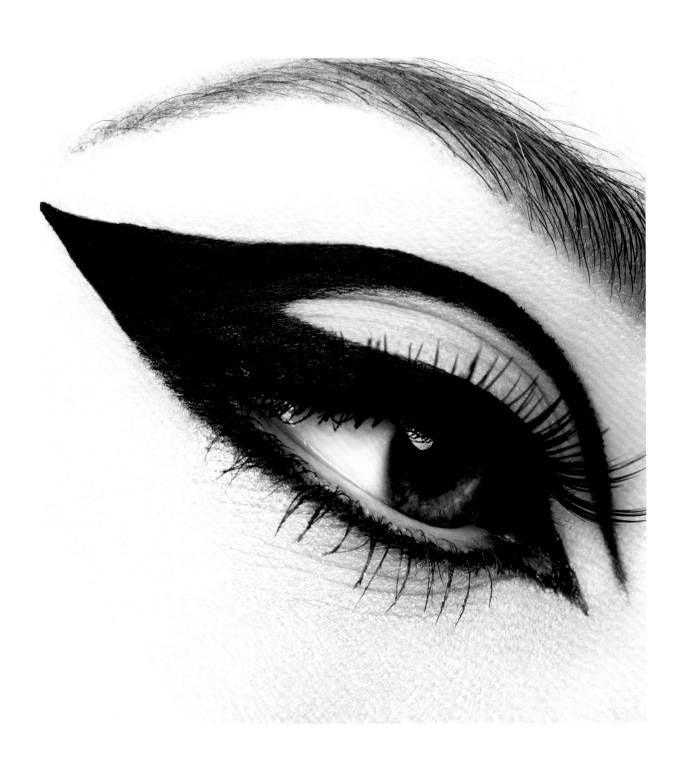

Makeup MAC Fluidline (Blacktrack),
Chromagraph Pencil (Pure White), Eye
Shadow (White Frost), Zoom Lash, 2 Lash
eyelashes **Photography** Catherine Harbour

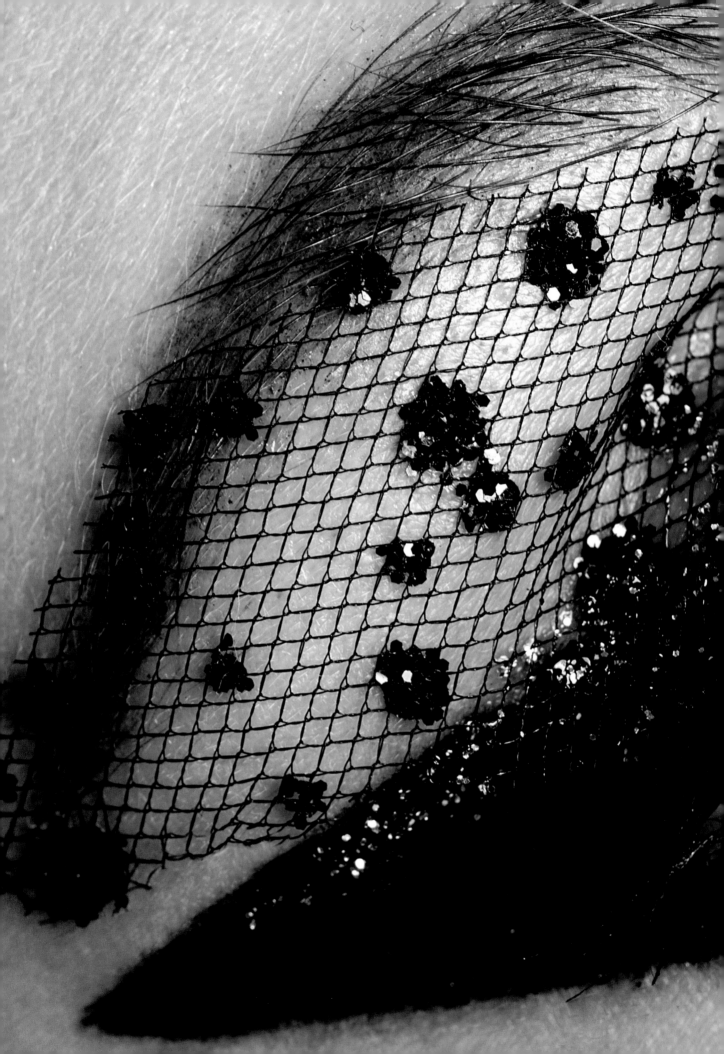

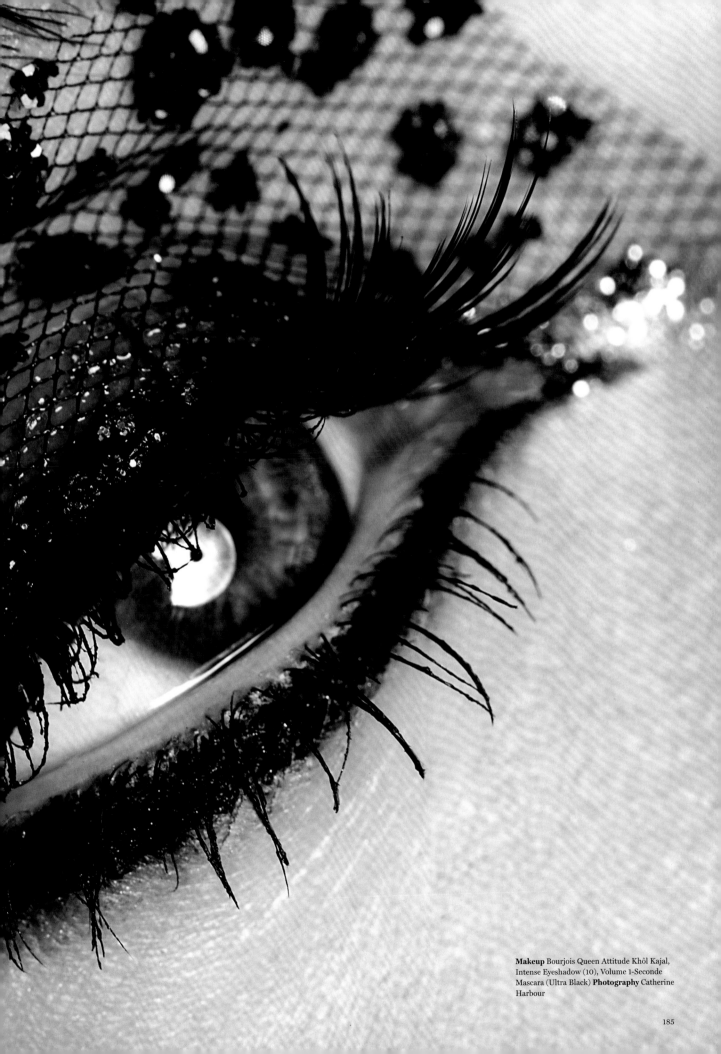

Makeup Bourjois Queen Attitude Khôl Kajal, Intense Eyeshadow (10), Volume 1-Seconde Mascara (Ultra Black) **Photography** Catherine Harbour

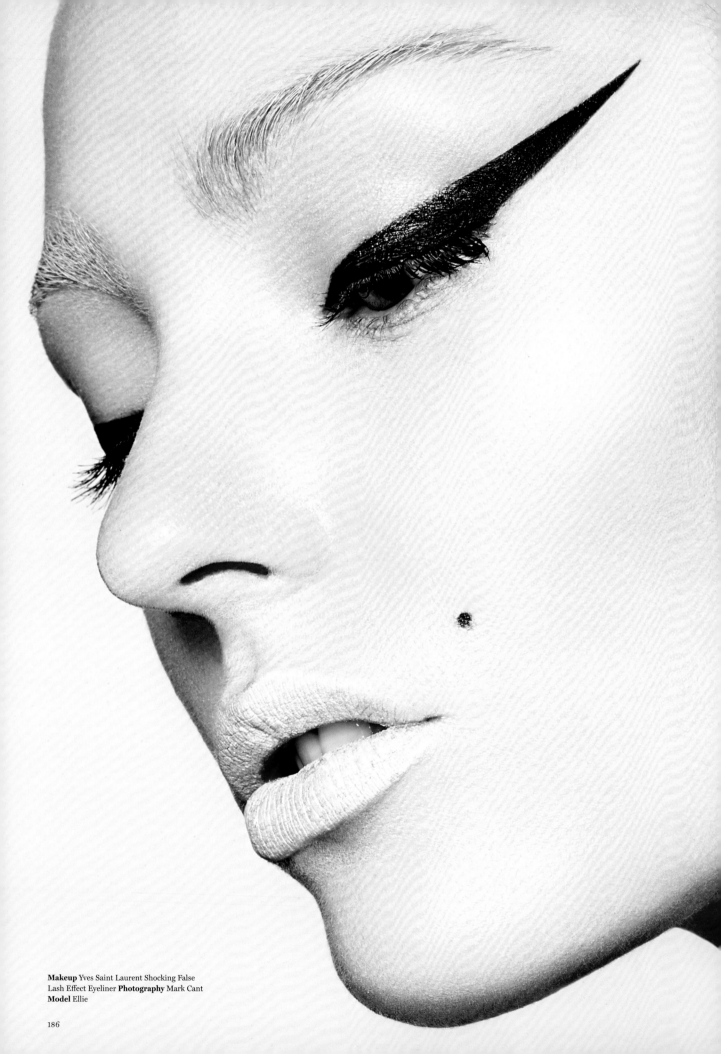

Makeup Yves Saint Laurent Shocking False
Lash Effect Eyeliner **Photography** Mark Cant
Model Ellie

Ideas for lined eyes

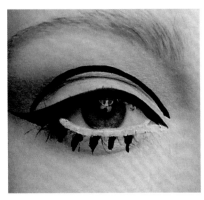

Max Factor Masterpiece Glide & Define
Liquid Eyeliner

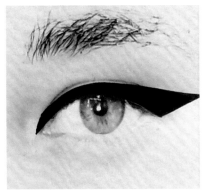

Yves Saint Laurent Shocking False Lash
Effect Eyeliner

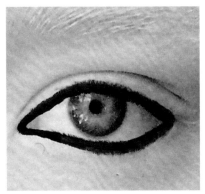

Bourjois Queen Attitude Khôl Kajal

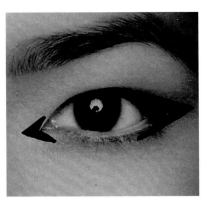

Bourjois Mega Liner

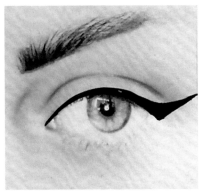

Rimmel Glam'Eyes

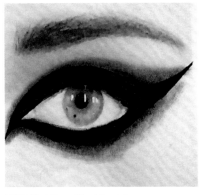

MAC Fluidline (Blacktrack)

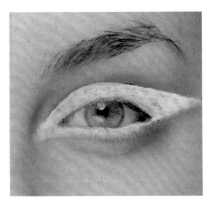

MAC Chromagraph Pencil (PureWhite)

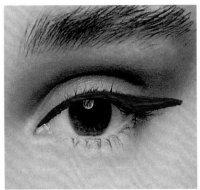

Yves Saint Laurent Dessin Du Regard Eye
Pencil no. 13

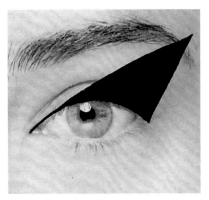

Barry M Wink Marker Pen

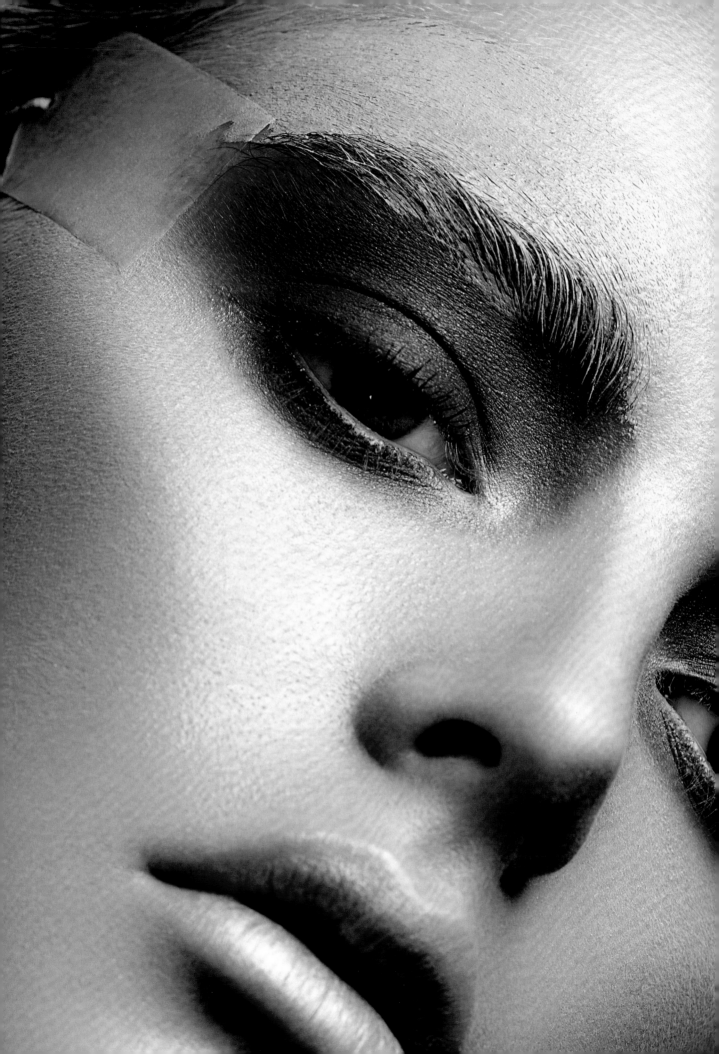

'I don't really believe in rules about colour on the eyes; it's the tone and shade that matter.'

Colour on the eyes

If you're overwhelmed by the rainbow of hues and textural finishes on the market, then blending a few shades of the same colour to add depth to the eye is a great place to start. On the whole, those with blue eyes should choose shades of taupe, brown, gold, plum, bronze and peach. Brown eyes can pull off a richer variety of shades, including neons, neutrals and metallics. Green eyes look beautiful with a swoop of purple or violet. The darkest shades should be worked into the eyelid crease and outer corner of the eye, with the palest hue at the inner corner.

Applying glitter can be a messy process, so make sure you have a good eyeshadow base to begin with, such as a greasepaint formula. Press the glitter into the eye paint with your finger so that it takes hold – a brush isn't always firm enough. A colourless wax-based product will make a brilliant mixing medium here.

In your technicolour beauty quest, don't neglect false eyelashes. Placed strategically, they add fullness and drama. Use packs of individual lashes to create a truly customized effect, layering them strategically – lengthen round eyes with longer lashes in the outer corner, or widen narrow eyes with airily light, curled lashes. For festivals, use glitter, feathers and stick-on body jewels to fine-tune your own carnival lash-look.

Makeup Mark Traynor FaceLift, Kryolan Supracolor Shimmering Vision Palette, Supracolor Interferenz Palette 6 Colors Duo-Chrome **Photography** Camille Sanson **Model** Sophie H @ Profile

Ideas for coloured eyes

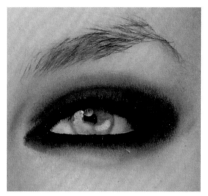

Tom Ford Eye Colour Quad (Titanium Smoke)

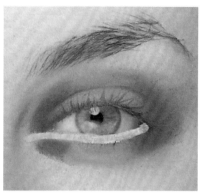

Kiko Water Eyeshadows (223, Eggplant Purple; 217, Mandarin); MAC Eye Kohl (Fascinating)

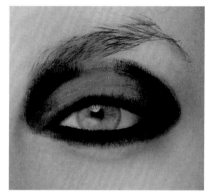

Barry M Metallic Eyeliner (mle4); MAC Eye Kohl (Smolder), Eye Shadow (Carbon)

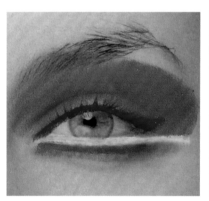

The Body Shop Colour Crush Eyeshadow (310, Berry Cheeky); NYX Eye Pencil (White)

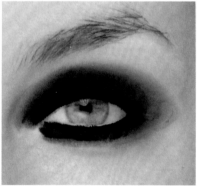

MAC Fluidline (Blacktrack); The Body Shop Colour Crush Eyeshadow (515, Blue Over You); MAC Eye Kohl (Smolder)

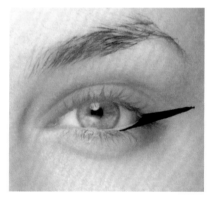

NARS Duo Eyeshadow (Rated R); Rimmel Glam'Eyes Liner

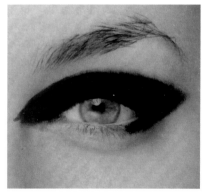

NARS Eye Paints (Snake Eyes, Iskandar)

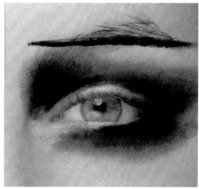

Make Up Store Cybershadow (Rumble), MAC Blacktrack; MAC Eye Shadows (Sketch, Plum Dressing, Gesso)

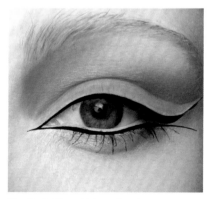

The Body Shop Colour Crush Eyeshadows (001, Sugar Glaze; 110, Sand By Me; 505 Boyfriend Jeans; 510, Something Blue; 601, Chat-Up-Lime; 605, Sweet Pea); Liquid Eyeliner (Black)

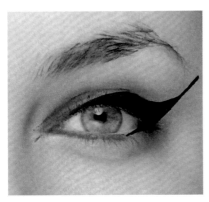

Make Up For Ever Aqua Cream (12, Golden Copper); MAC Fluidline (Blacktrack)

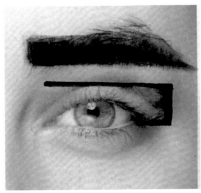

The Body Shop Colour Crush Eyeshadow (240 Gorgeous Gold), Liquid Eyeliner

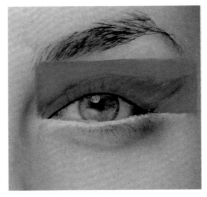

Kryolan HD Cream Liners (Sweet Pink, Ocean)

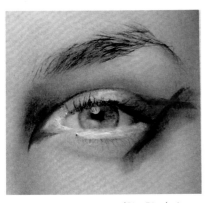

Kryolan HD Cream Liner (Sky Blue), Aqua and Night Blue from the Shades Eye Shadow Palette (Dublin)

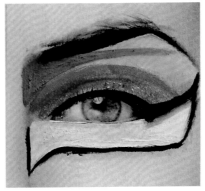

Make Up For Ever 12 Flash Color Case

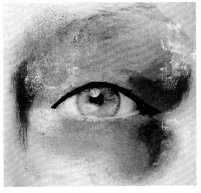

Kryolan Supracolor Shimmering Vision Palette

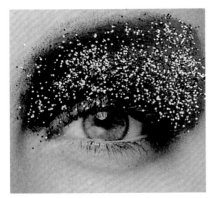

Make Up For Ever 12 Flash Color Case; MAC Glitter (3D Silver)

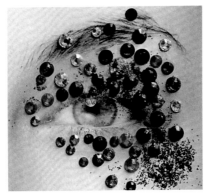

Kryolan eye colours in Pink and Swarovski Crystals

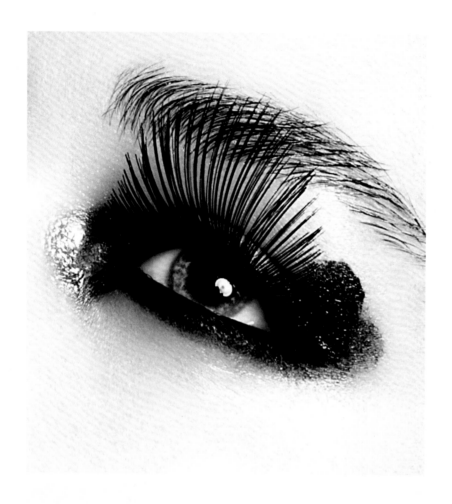

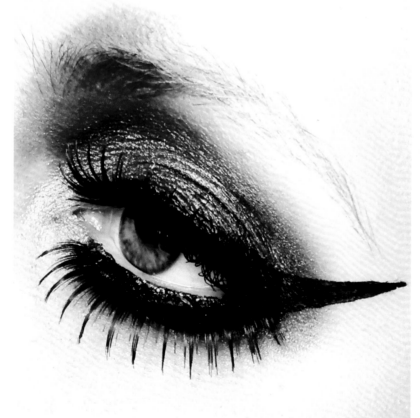

Above **Makeup** MAC Eye Kohl
(Smolder), Glitters (Turquoise, 3D
Black); Eldora eyelashes

Left **Makeup** MAC Lashes, Glitters
(Amber Lights, Chrome Yellow,
Cranberry, Reflects Antique Gold,
Reflects Bronze), Eye Kohl (Smolder)

Opposite **Makeup** MAC Pigments
(Deep Blue Green, Golden Olive);
Eldora eyelashes **Photography** Camille
Sanson **Model** Zoey Kay

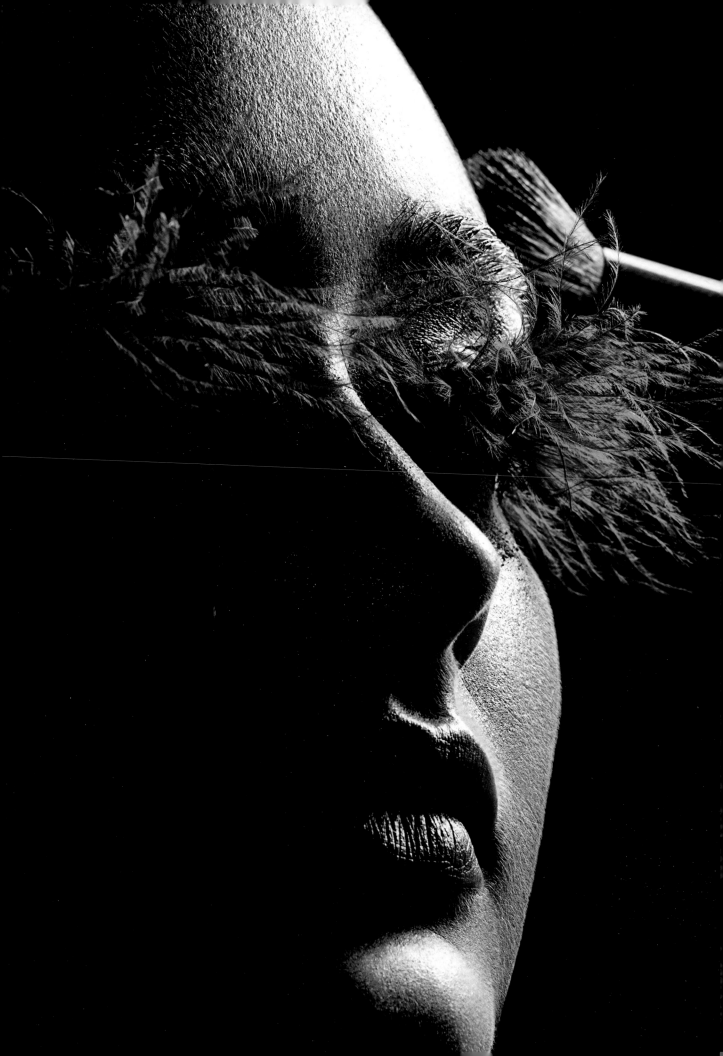

Get the look

Having the right brushes is essential – they should be considered an extension of your hand. Every result is dependent on pressure and movement, and over time brushes are moulded into the shape of how you use them to apply makeup. These are my basic essentials.

Tools of the trade
Clockwise from centre-top

1. MOXI 01 Taklon Foundation Brush

2. MAC 208 Angled Brow Brush

3. The Body Shop Eyeshadow Blender Brush

4. Kryolan Professional Fan Brush

5. Shu Uemura Synthetic Brush 6m

6. Hakuhodo Powder Blush Brush

7. Charles Fox Concealer Brush

8. Shu Uemura Powder Brush (158)

9. Make Up For Ever Bronzing and Contour Brush

10. Kryolan Premium Eyeshadow Brush 9363 (used for nose contour and highlights)

11. Charles Fox Cheekbone Contour Brush

12. MAC 233 Highlighter Brush for Cream

13. Shu Uemura Eyeshadow Placement Brush no.10

14. Charles Fox Socket Blender 681479

15. MAC 239 Highlighter and Brow Bone Blender

Photography Catherine Harbour **Model** Zoe Banks @ MOT Models

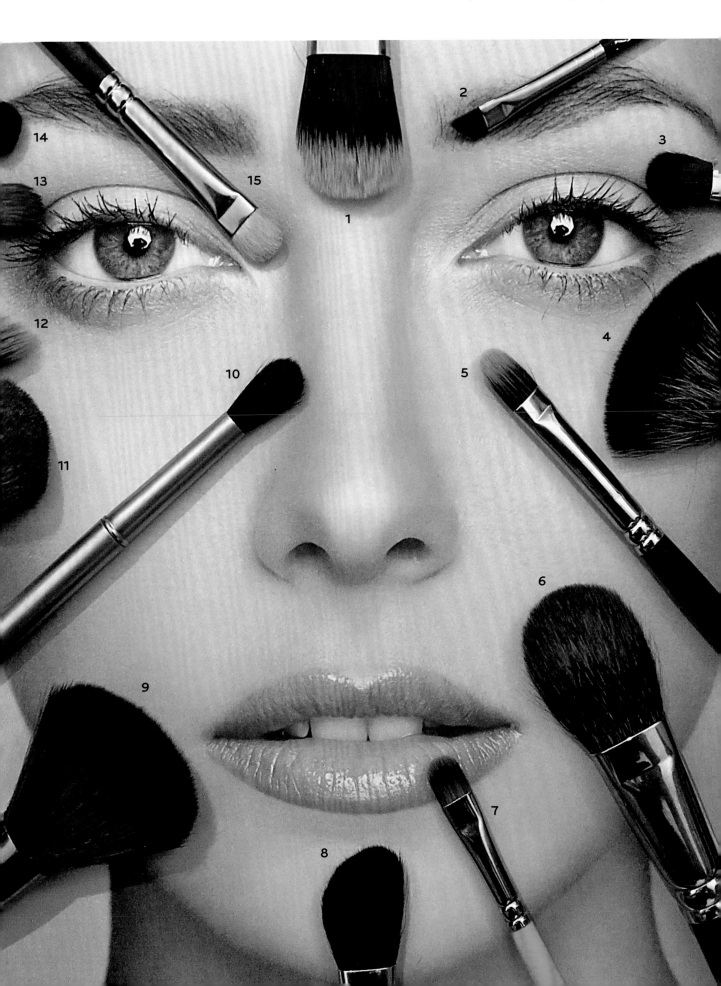

Creating a dramatic smoky eye on smaller-lidded eyes

Smoky eyes are a classic look that can work well on all eye shapes. Clever use of colour and shading makes the eyes look wider, more intense and bigger, but also balances eye shapes that are perhaps not symmetrical. Once a basic technique is applied it is easy to adapt the look. Creating a smoky look on smaller eyes produces a smouldering and intense effect – making them look bigger and wider can create a beautifully dramatic look.

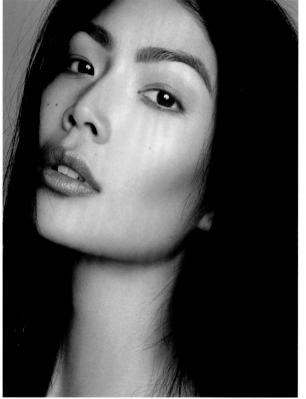 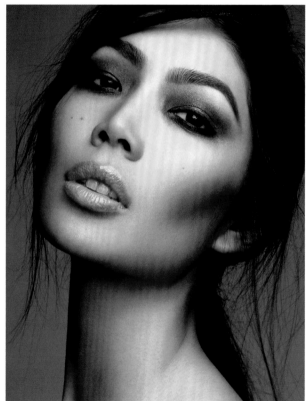

Skin is prepped with Benefit PORfessional, That Gal Brightening Face Primer. Brows groomed with Tweezerman tweezers and Browmousse **Photography** Catherine Harbour **Hair** Chie Sato using Label.m **Model** Angie

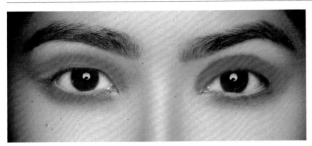

Step 1
Create base with Armani Face Fabric Foundation, NARS Concealer, Laura Mercier Secret Brightening Powder and The Body Shop Brow & Lash Gel.

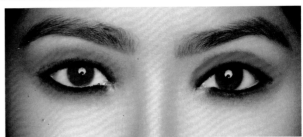

Step 2
Apply Make Up For Ever Aqua Cream (12, Golden Copper) all over lid to the socket line following eye shape.

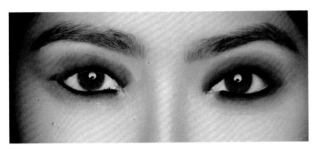

Step 3
Add MAC Eye Pencil (Smolder) to inner rim on top and bottom of water line and smudge into lash line.

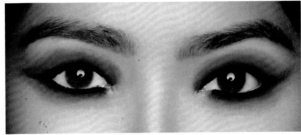

Step 4
Use NARS Duo Eyeshadow (Isolde) to darken inner eye area up to start of eyebrows and under-eye areas with the gold. Darken sockets with the brown.

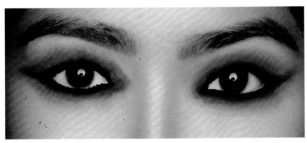

Step 5
Reapply eye pencil on the lash line creating a winged line, and smudge around lash line and outwards to fade.

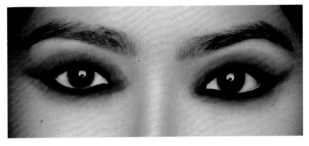

Step 6
Intense and smudge edges with NARS Duo Eyeshadow (Surabaya) and wing out. Build up and smudge under eye, connecting the inner corners.

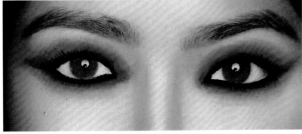

Step 7
Add Giorgio Armani Maestro Eyeliner and finish with Bourjois Beauty'Full Volume Dark Khôl Mascara on top and bottom lashes. Shade and contour with MAC Sculpting Powder Pro Palette (Sculpt, Shadester) on the bone, and fade to hairline; also include the sides of the nose.

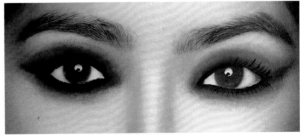

Step 8
Highlight down the centre of the nose and above cheekbones with MAC Eye Shadow (White Frost). Nude out lips with MAC Lipstick (Peachstock) and finish with a touch of Lustreglass (Instant Gold).

Creating a dramatic smoky look on big eyes

Creating smoky eyes on bigger, wide eyes is all about definition and graduation. The application can be a lot softer and still be dramatic. There is lots of space to add shadow with bigger eyes, but the secret is to control the look so it balances eye shapes on the face.

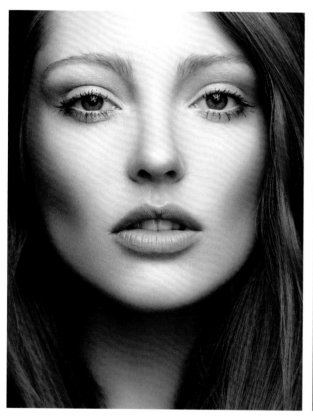

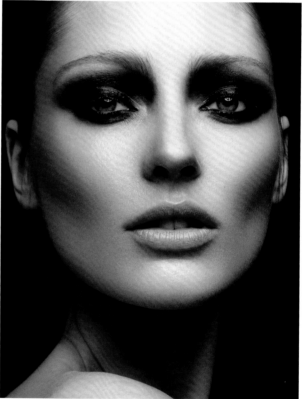

Skin is prepped with Benefit PORfessional, That Gal Brightening Face Primer. Brows groomed with Tweezerman tweezers and Browmousse **Photography** Catherine Harbour **Hair** Chie Sato using Label.m **Model** Ellie

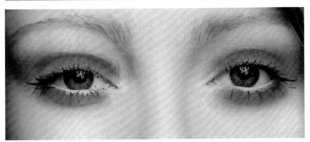

Step 1
Create base with YSL Top Secrets All-In-One BB Cream, The Body Shop Radiant Highlighter and NARS Concealer. Apply MAC Eye Shadow (Bronze) under eye and all over lid to socket.

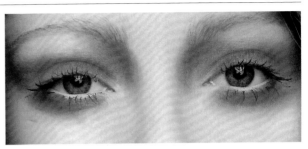

Step 2
Brush on Laura Mercier Illuminating Eye Colour (Earth Glow) in sockets and blend towards nose outline and under beginning of brow. Sweep underneath eye to darken near lash line.

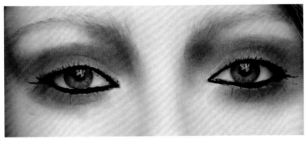

Step 3
Use Giorgio Armani Eyes to Kill Solo (3) in sockets and blend to inner eye by nose. Apply Yves Saint Laurent Eye Pencil (Velvet Black) in the inner water line and smudge.

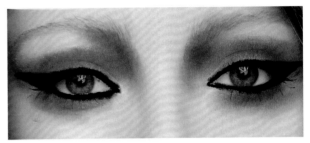

Step 4
Reapply eye pencil on the top lash line and wing out.

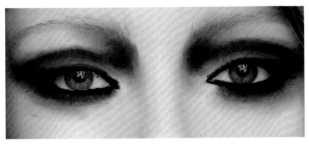

Step 5
Join the corners and blend out in sockets, inner eye to brow and underneath lash line using MAC Eye Shadow (Carbon).

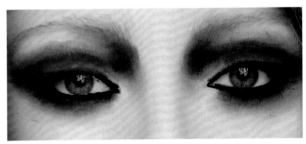

Step 6
Add MAC Eye Shadow (Plum Dressing) in the middle of the lid and blend on the edges under eye and sockets.

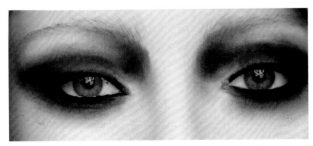

Step 7
Create a strong winged liner along the top lash line using Lancôme Artliner in black. Apply plenty of Yves Saint Laurent Shocking Mascara (Deep Black).

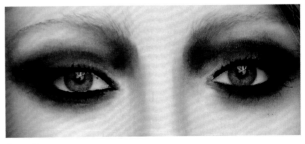

Step 8
Highlight inner eye with MAC Eye Shadow (White Frost), contour cheekbones with Sculpting Powder Pro Palette (Shadester). Apply NARS Velvet Matte Lip Pencil (Roman Holiday).

Creating the Renoir-inspired oil-painting look

To recreate this look it is important to have a variety of soft brushes, as every stroke you create has a different colour. Always remember that there is no right or wrong – you must just feel that it works. Be free and choose whatever colours you like.

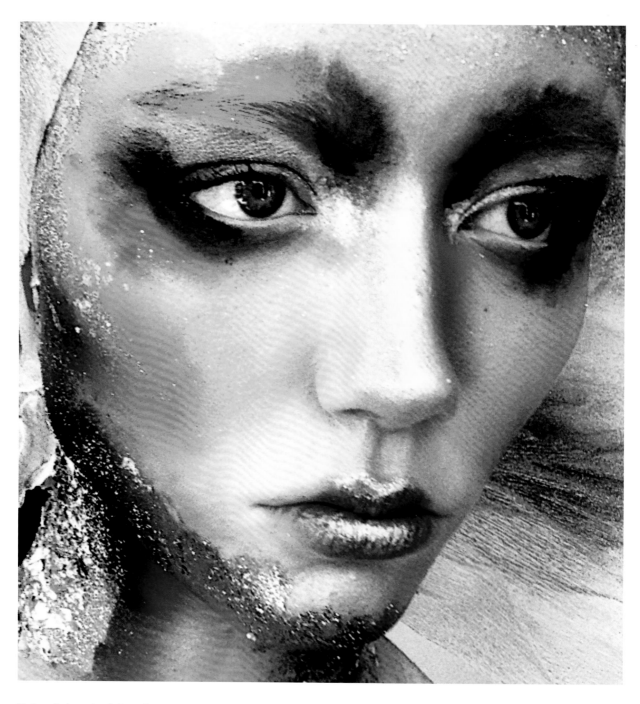

Photography image above by Lan on her iPhone, step-by-step images by Lolo Creative
Model Claudia @ Premier

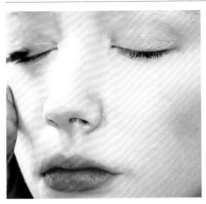

Step 1
Apply yellow greasepaint on the eyelid, stopping at the socket line.

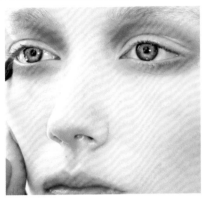

Step 2
Using a soft brush, apply neon pink into the socket, blending upwards to the brow in a circular motion, fading away to the outer brow. Blend a line under the eyes.

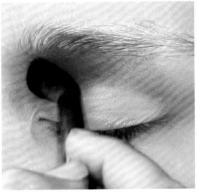

Step 3
Add a darker colour such as purple in the inner socket to the brow, where the nose meets it.

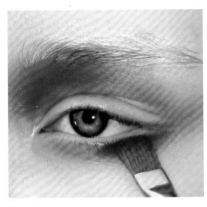

Step 4
Add a darker colour such as purple on the outer, lower under-eye.

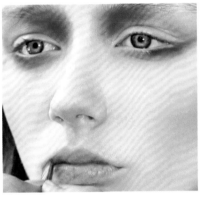

Step 5
Fill in the lips and cheeks with pale pink. Next, apply orange greasepaint using a bigger brush to the centre of the T-zone areas and centre of the neck.

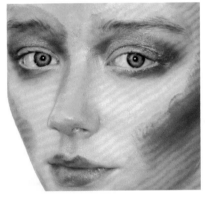

Step 6
Reapply the pink and darker purple to contour and blend into the cheeks. Top up the yellow on the lids and set with a powder metallic glitter or eye shadow.

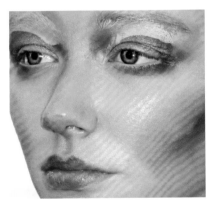

Step 7
Using pale blue and purple greasepaint, layer on from the nose to the eye sockets and add a layer of pale pink on the cheeks. Add another layer of darker pink on lips.

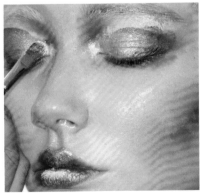

Step 8
Use iridescent reflecting powder in gold or white shimmer and place in the inner eye and centre of lips for extra highlights. Place down the centre of the nose.

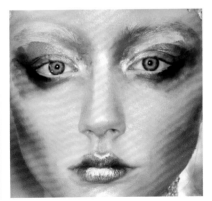

Step 9
Use black greasepaint at the bottom outer-eye corners and smudge; when it mixes with pink and purple, dark blue emerges. Finish with gold leaf sparsely placed around the hairline and neck.

Creating the Henry Moore-inspired graphic look

Creating a look that's not symmetrical can be daunting. Here balance is key, learning to play with highlights on the bone structure. Following the jaw line and creating shadows helps to maintain balance. Practise building up the layers and learn to judge when is enough; there are no particular rules to follow.

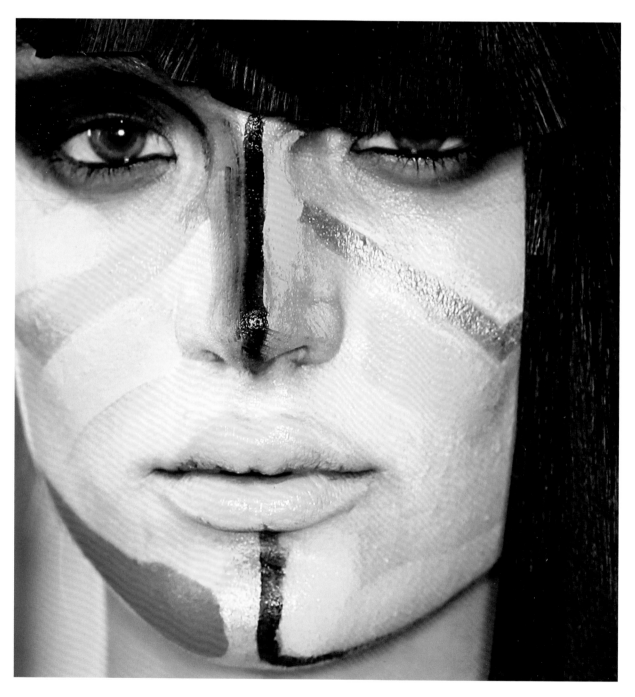

Photography Camille Sanson **Hair** Diana Moar **Model** Mimi

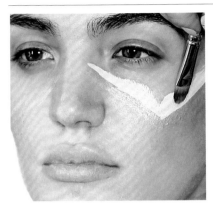

Step 1
Use white from the Make Up For Ever 12 Flash Color Case to outline a V-shape across nose to cheek and hairline.

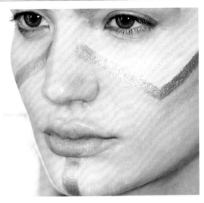

Step 2
Repeat underneath the same line using the gold metallic greasepaint colour and add to the centre of the chin.

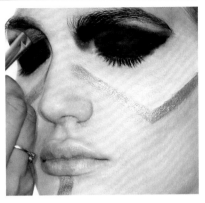

Step 3
Use The Bodyshop Colour Crush Eyeshadow (015, Moonlight Kiss) to blend all over the eye socket; smudge into the inner brow and blend away.

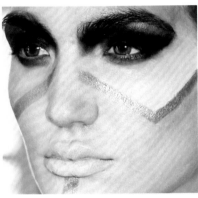

Step 4
Use MAC Eye Shadow (Bronze) under eye and edge of black to blend away. Add MAC Eye Shadow (White Frost) to highlight inner corner of eye and use white greasepaint to make it solid.

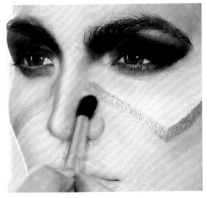

Step 5
Go over foundation with MAC Full Coverage Foundation (W10). Use the White Frost eyeshadow to set area above cheekbone, and translucent powder to mattify skin.

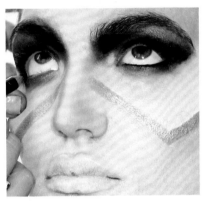

Step 6
Add MAC Eye Kohl (Smolder) to inner water line and smudge into lashes.

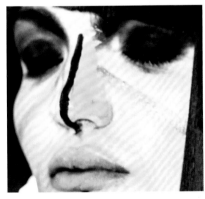

Step 7
Using black greasepaint colours from the palette, outline the centre of the nose.

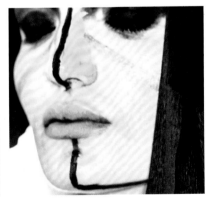

Step 8
Outline the chin and map the jaw line on one side of the face.

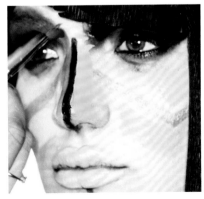

Step 9
Use the purple, blue, yellow and pink from the greasepaint palette to shade and block on lips, cheeks and eyes. Finish with more colour, feel free to experiment.

Afterword

Before I began my career, I would not have believed that I would be working as a makeup artist today and still enjoying it. I believe that the ups and downs have all been important lessons in my growth in this industry, and have prepared me for the bigger opportunities that could change my life. I may have been naïve to think that everyone would want to help me, but it turns out that sometimes not everyone wants you to do well. Some will work harder than others, some are lucky that they know the right people, and some are just in the right place at the right time. The most important thing is to be open and grateful for any opportunity and to learn from that experience. Surround yourself with people who love you and support you.

Ultimately, I have been challenged throughout my career and fortunate that I have been able to learn from my experiences. At times I was close to giving it all up. I'm glad now that I have stuck with my instincts and carried on, otherwise I would not be sharing my story today. One job has always led to another, and that is exciting because it means that every day is different. Word of mouth is the most important PR for a makeup artist.

I enjoy working on live shows, which are one of the most exciting parts of the fashion and beauty industry. It is challenging because there are so many aspects to be aware of, such as designing months before a show, testing the look and researching to make sure it's fashion forward for the next season. You learn to work as a team and to strict deadlines: there are other things to be done such as dress fittings, run-throughs, hair and nails, and sometimes the late arrivals of models. There is no time for mistakes or retouching – it is live, which is why placement and perfection is the key. Being self-motivated and calm under pressure are essential skills to have. The reward is when the final results are on the catwalk for everyone to see and this makes it all worthwhile.

Taking inspiration from shows and what is happening in the industry enables me to have fun and be creative on photoshoots. I put everything I learn into practice. Testing with photographers is great for improving technique and portfolio work. It is important to feel inspired when working on everyday jobs, so by working on my own shoots it gives me the creative outlet I need. I learn so much from my team and am very lucky to have found talented creatives who share the same vision as me. It is so important to have a good working relationship as it creates a great environment to work in and it's easy to share ideas. It's always good to work with people who are better than you as you can learn more, elevating your work to the next level.

One challenge can be working with famous talent, as your job as a makeup artist goes beyond being about what you can learn. No longer is it an anonymous model who sits in your chair and leaves when you're finished – this is a person who can never be off-guard. I love working with celebrities as it's like having a peek into someone's life while making him or her happy. Being responsible for their image can be a full-time job, following their every step through the working day. Being a good listener and a friend, being confident, reliable and calm are just some of the traits that are essential in building a relationship with a celebrity. Striving to be the best at all times and knowledgeable about trends is important in keeping the look current. Often celebrities will have their own look, which needs to be maintained and tweaked. They are recognized around the world not only for their talent but also for their image.

In music and film the hours are really long and repetitive. The important things about working on a set are teamwork and deadlines. Once the makeup is done it's all about maintaining the look so it's perfect at all times. Character work can take up to six hours to create when special effects are included, so it is important to know of the best products available as this can make life easier. There are many elements to understand, especially in film, which might have numerous different locations to consider and will not be limited to a studio shoot. On location, makeup has to withstand weather conditions, while dealing with underwater makeup is another skill altogether. Some artists do specialize in particular areas, but I love it all so I try to work on as many interesting productions as I can.

Being a makeup artist means being a self-contained business, and this is something I have learnt late in my career. With all of the hands-on experience and knowledge that I have gained, without realizing it I have become a business and my name is my brand. In order to succeed and advance to the next level, having a mentor or agent is essential because they deal with all the bookings and can open many doors. Working behind the scenes all the time, it's easy to forget about putting yourself forward. It's scary, but those feelings are the same as feeling excited – you never know what's around the corner.

Understanding the needs of others is truly key to getting the look right. It is instinct to know the difference between beautiful and ugly, right and wrong. Every brushstroke makes that change and creates a signature look. You can teach techniques to a certain degree, but you can't teach how someone should precisely create a look. I believe you feel it. There is an emotional attachment to every look I create, and I hope that I evoke this feeling of beauty and inspiration within everyone I work with.

Lan Nguyen-Grealis

Contributors

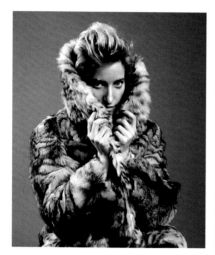

Hannah Kane, Writer and Editor
www.phoenixmag.co.uk

Hannah is the Editor-in-Chief of *PHOENIX*, a magazine available worldwide, representing London's vibrant fashion and culture scene. After studying Human Rights Law, Hannah completed a postgraduate certificate in Fashion and Lifestyle Journalism at the London College of Fashion. She has written for a variety of media including *Time Out London*, CNN, *The Daily Rubbish*, *Disorder* and *Shiny Media*, before editing *The GFW Daily*, *Fashionista Magazine* and TheFashionScout.com. She has also worked as a branding and PR consultant to several major consumer retailers.

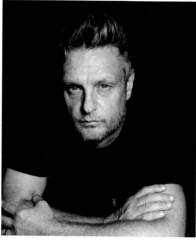

Rankin, Photographer
www.rankin.co.uk

Rankin is an internationally acclaimed British portrait and fashion photographer and filmmaker. After co-founding *Dazed & Confused* in 1991 he went on to publish his own fashion magazine *RANK*, followed by *AnOther Magazine* and *Hunger*. An Honorary Fellow of the Royal Photographic Society, he has published numerous books as well as working on films, music videos and commercials. Based in London, Rankin continues to work with those at the cutting edge of fashion, music, the arts and culture.

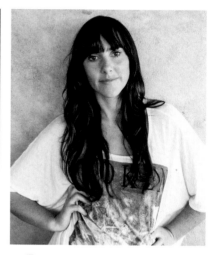

Camille Sanson, Photographer
www.camilesanson.com

Camille is a London-based photographer from New Zealand. She has worked with publications including *Tatler*, *Elle* and *Glamour*, cosmetics brands such as L'Oreal and Yves Saint Laurent, and fashion labels including Karen Walker and Finery London. She also works with technology companies producing advertising and photographic campaigns for brands such as Orange/EE and HTC. Lan and Camille met in 2004 at London Fashion Week and quickly formed a creative friendship. Soon after they started collaborating, striving to push the boundaries and progress their own distinctive styles.

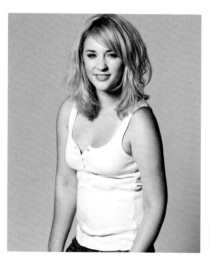

Catherine Harbour, Photographer
www.catherineharbour.com

Catherine is a London-based photographer with a wealth of experience shooting fashion, beauty and advertising around the world. She has photographed campaigns for M&S, USC, East, Republic, Simply Yours, Pink Sands, Damsel and Burlington Arcade, and her work has featured in top fashion magazines including *Cosmopolitan*, *Esquire*, *InStyle*, *JFW*, *OK!*, *S Magazine*, and *Look*. She was nominated for Fashion Photographer of the Year 2010, and has contributed to recent series of Britain and Ireland's Next Top Model with Thumbs Up Productions.

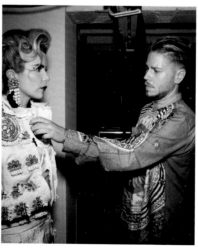

Karl Willett, Celebrity Stylist
www.karlwillett.co.uk

Known for his elegant yet contemporary style, Karl has achieved a distinguished international clientele. As a self-taught stylist, his career began in the window display team at Selfridges & Co, London, and he has since become a much sought-after stylist and creative director. Karl's ability to re-brand clients has secured him a formidable reputation within the entertainment industry. He has a broad portfolio, ranging from fashion and editorial styling to art direction and artist image consultancy. Karl has featured as a style expert on BBC Radio 1, and guest lecturer at Condé Nast College of Fashion & Design in London.

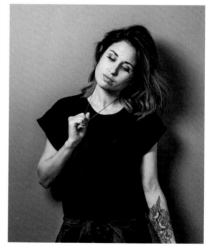

Diana Moar, Hairstylist
www.dianamoar.com

Diana began her hairdressing career over 12 years ago and was successful from a young age. After winning countless awards in her home country of New Zealand she moved to London, where she has quickly risen through the ranks. Her broad skill set has given her the opportunity to work with some of the most celebrated photographers, stylists and publications. Known for her inventive and conceptual skills, she cuts, styles, colours and creates. Diana's passion is for session hair styling, and her longstanding creative collaborations allow her to continue working in this, the field that she loves.

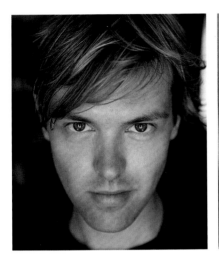

John Oakley, Photographer
www.oakleyphotography.co.uk

An international fashion and campaign photographer, John is currently based in London, freelancing and enjoying working with celebrities and collaborating with like-minded creatives. John's passion for detail and love for his clients' concepts takes him on many interesting projects on locations worldwide. He has worked for clients including *PHOENIX*, *EM Magazine*, *Idoll Magazine* and Tresor Paris.

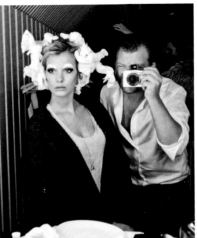

Mark Cant, Photographer
www.markcant.com

Mark lives and works in London shooting fashion, beauty and celebrities for a wide range of high profile magazines including *Wonderland*, *Cosmopolitan* and *i-D*. Known for his striking images and portraits of his characters, there is a distinctive energy in his work.

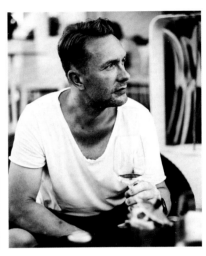

Gary Nunn, Photographer
www.garynunn.co.uk

Gary was born in the outskirts of London in 1978, and his obsession with people, creativity, detail and subsequently photography started early. Being self taught and taking inspiration from many different sources has enabled him to create a notable editorial and theatrical style with a swoosh of glamour. He has been lucky enough to carve out striking imagery from limited opportunities, working with talented international teams. His work has featured in publications including *GQ Magazine*, *Vogue Italia* and *Grazia*.

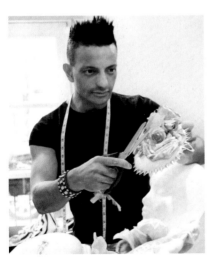

Louis Mariette, Couture Milliner
www.louismariette.com

Iconic creator of extraordinary headpieces, Louis lives in the bubble of his endless imagination. A passionate artist, he is also a great believer in supporting others. He is vice-president of The Children's Trust and runs marathons for them, has trekked to the summit of Kilimanjaro, is Patron of St Thomas Lupus Trust, and supports Survival International. He makes regular appearances in the media and co-hosted the BBC's celebration coverage of Royal Ascot's 300th year, was a judge on series 5 of Britain's Next Top Model, and has appeared in Four Rooms on Channel 4.

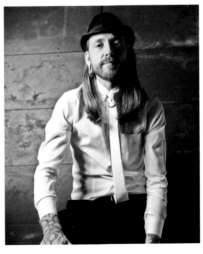

Justin Smith, Couture Milliner
www.jsmithesquire.com

Justin began his couture millinery label J Smith Esquire following the critical acclaim of his 2007 graduation show at London's Royal College of Art. He alternates creating his own collections and exhibiting at fashion's most prestigious international events with collaborations for high-end designers like Stella McCartney and such iconic film work as Angelina Jolie's Maleficent horned headdress, as well as bespoke commissions and one-off showpieces. Examples of his incredible couture millinery are with private collectors and museums the world over, including London's V&A and FIT in New York.

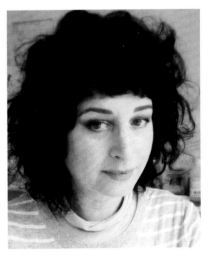

Phyllis Cohen, MD of Face•Lace
www.face-lace.com

Phyllis has always used her illustration background in her makeup. She has worked for publications including *Vogue*, *Vanity Fair*, *Tatler* and *Dazed & Confused*, and with celebrities such as David Bowie, Annie Lennox and Daphne Guinness. Her exceptional body painting has featured in many advertising campaigns. She has an MA in Fine Art from the renowned Goldsmiths College, where she researched makeup science. In 2012, Phyllis launched the cult brand Face•Lace, intricate ready-to-wear makeup designs and facial adornments, now sold in 16 countries worldwide.

Acknowledgments

I want to thank my team and everyone who has collaborated with me to help bring my vision to life, especially my friend and photographer Camille Sanson: you have been there from the beginning of my career and helped me to take it to another level. Your help and support have been invaluable. I have learnt so much, and you have helped me in my journey to become a better artist and educator by creating this book. I thank you from the bottom of my heart for sharing this journey with me. You inspire me.

To Catherine Harbour and Karl Willett: huge thanks for always understanding my ideas, no matter how crazy they sound, but most of all for being true friends.

To Hannah Kane, for helping me to write this book and communicate all my ideas and inspirations with words that I couldn't have done without. Your input has been invaluable.

Thank you to all of my friends who have stood by me during the hard times and encouraged me to carry on, with your loyalty and positive advice, through the difficult times. Thanks especially to my parents, who have allowed me to follow my dreams and to be who I am, and to my brothers and sisters for their support and for always being there for me in life and work.

Thank you to Wolfram Langer, Dominik Langer, Nadine Langer, Ann Lee, Vitoria Lee, and Paul Merchant especially for believing in my work, and thanks to all the team at Kryolan and Charles Fox Ltd for the continued support and opportunities that have allowed me to grow in ways I never thought possible.

Thank you to Laurence King Publishing, especially to Sophie Drysdale and Gaynor Sermon, for bringing this book to life and helping it to achieve its full potential.

A special thanks to Rankin for taking time out from his busy schedule, for his vision and kind words in the foreword.

Thank you to Paloma Faith, a strong woman and icon, for your kind words, wisdom, and especially support.

Very many thanks to Tuuli Shipster, Lolo Creative, Pebbles Akins, Zaida Ibrahim-Gani, Yuko Fredrikkson, Indigo Rohrer, Kelly Mendiola, Yelena Konnova, Eoin Whelan, Kerry White, Alexa Taylor, Jay Gill, Selina Davis, Ivana Nohel, Marc Eastlake, Klare Wilkinson, James Langon, Jose Quijano, Chie Sato, Sacha Mascolo-Tarbuck and Toni & Guy, Carlos Conteras, Rua Acorn, Phyllis Cohen, Hannah Maestranzi, Joey Bevan, Gary Nunn, Adele Pentland, Vivian Nwonka, Louis Mariette, Justin Smith, Daniel Lismore, William Tempest, Jessica Bumpus, Kimberly Wyatt, Daniel Sandler, Rachel Wood, Sandra Cooke, Lianna Fouler, Amber Doyle, Russella, Nathalie Gayne, Attracta Courtney, Katrin Straupe and Charles Moriarty.

To the model agencies Storm, Select, Nevs, Profile, MOT and Lenis, thank you.

Thanks for the image retouching by Lucy Hutchinson.

Thank you to all the PRs of the cosmetics brands that have supported me through the years by supplying me with all of my favourite products, which I have used to create my looks, especially Zoe Cook, Lesley Chievers, Christina Aristodemou and Jo Scicluna.

To my husband Brendan Grealis, who is my best friend and rock, who has always protected me and given me the courage to not be afraid and to follow my dreams. Thank you. I am so grateful to have you in my life and for the arrival of our baby daughter Eva Marie – who was the motivation to complete this project. I dedicate this book to both of you.

Resources

Makeup-art trade shows and exhibitions
IMATS (International Make-up Artist Trade Show)
   International exhibitions held throughout the year
   www.imats.net
Make-Up Artist Design Show (MADS), Düsseldorf
   www.make-up-artist-show.com
Olympia Beauty, London, UK
   www.olympiabeauty.co.uk
Paintopia, UK www.paintopiafestival.com
Professional Beauty North, Manchester, UK
   www.professionalbeauty.co.uk
The Prosthetics Event, UK
   www.theprostheticsevent.co.uk
Salon International, UK www.salonexhibitions.co.uk
United Makeup Artist Expo (UMA), London, UK
   www.umae.co.uk
World Body Painting Festival (WBPF), Germany
   www.bodypainting-festival.com

Specialist suppliers
Kryolan www.kryolan.com
Charles Fox www.charlesfox.co.uk
Screenface www.screenface.co.uk
Guru Makeup Emporium Ltd
   www.gurumakeupemporium.com
PAM: Precious About Make-up Ltd
   www.preciousaboutmakeup.com
TILT Professional Makeup www.tiltmakeup.com

Credits

The author and publisher would like to thank everyone who contributed to this book. Photography and styling credits accompany each image within the book, with the addition of the following:
p26 © Succession Picasso/DACS, London 2015/White Images/Scala
p48 © The Estate of Alberto Giacometti (Fondation Giacometti, Paris and ADAGP, Paris), licensed in the UK by ACS and DACS, London 2015/Bridgeman Images.
p72 © 20th Century Fox/The Kobal Collection
p98 © Franco Fojanini/Getty Images